Amiloride and Epithelial Sodium Transport

Proceedings of a Symposium on Basic Mechanisms in Transporting
Epithelia Using Amiloride held at Valley Forge, Pennsylvania, April 7,
1978

Symposium on Basic Mechanisms in Transporting Epithelia Using Amiloride, Valley Forge, Pa., 1978.

Amiloride and Epithelial Sodium Transport

Edited by

Alan W. Cuthbert

Department of Pharmacology
University of Cambridge
Cambridge
UK

George M. Fanelli, Jr.

and

Alexander Scriabine

Merck Institute for Therapeutic Research
West Point, Pennsylvania
USA

Urban & Schwarzenberg • Baltimore-Munich 1979

Urban & Schwarzenberg, Inc.
7 E. Redwood Street
Baltimore, Maryland 21202
U.S.A.

Urban & Schwarzenberg
Pettenkoferstrasse 18
D-8000 München 2
GERMANY

Library of Congress Cataloging in Publication Data

Symposium on Basic Mechanisms in Transporting Epithelia
   Using Amiloride, Valley Forge, Pa., 1978.
   Amiloride and epithelial sodium transport.

   Includes index.
   1. Sodium metabolism—Congresses.   2. Biological
transport—Congresses.   3. Amiloride—Physiological
effect—Congresses.   4. Epithelium—Drug effects—
Congresses.   I. Cuthbert, Alan William.   II. Fanelli,
George M.   III. Scriabine, Alexander.   IV. Title
[DNLM: 1. Pyrazines—Pharmacodynamics—Congresses.
2. Epithelium—Metabolism—Congresses.   3. Biological
transport—Drug effects—Congresses.   4. Sodium—
Metabolism—Congresses.

QV95 S978a 1978 (P)]
QP535.N2S95 1978   79-251   591.1′858

ISBN   0-8067-0311-3   (Baltimore)
ISBN   3-541-70311-3   (München)

Printed in the United States of America

Table of Contents

Editors

Alan W. Cuthbert
Department of Pharmacology
University of Cambridge
Hills Road
Cambridge
UK

George M. Fanelli, Jr.
Senior Investigator
Renal Pharmacology
Merck Institute for Therapeutic
    Research
West Point, PA 19486 USA

Alexander Scriabine
Executive Director, Pharmacology
Biological Research
Merck Institute for Therapeutic
    Research
West Point, PA 19486 USA

Participants

J. Aceves
Department of Pharmacology
University of Cambridge
Hills Road
Cambridge
UK

E. v. Arnim
Physiologisches Institut der
    Universität München
Pettenkoferstrasse 12
D-8000 München 2
West Germany

R. Bauer
Physiologisches Institut der
    Universität München
Pettenkoferstrasse 12
D-8000 München 2
West Germany

P. J. Bentley
Department of Pharmacology
Mt. Sinai School of Medicine
100th Street and Fifth Avenue
New York, NY 10029 USA

Thomas U. L. Biber
Medical College of Virginia
Richmond, VA 23298 USA

John D. Biggers
Department of Physiology and
    Laboratory of Human
    Reproduction and Reproductive
    Biology
Harvard Medical School
Boston, MA 02115 USA

David W. Cochran
Merck, Sharp & Dohme Research
    Laboratories
West Point, PA 19486 USA

J. Crabbé
Departments of Physiology and
    Medicine
University of Louvain (U.C.L.)
    Medical School
Brussels
Belgium

Edward J. Cragoe, Jr.
Merck, Sharp & Dohme Research
Laboratories
West Point, PA 19486 USA

D. Cremaschi
Instituto di Fisologia Generale
Universita di Bori
Via Amendola 165/A
Bari
Italy

A. Dörge
Physiologisches Institut der
Universität München
Pettenkoferstrasse 12
D-8000 München 2
West Germany

W. Van Driessche
Laboratorium voor Fysiology
Universiteit te Leuven
Belgium

M. J. Edwardson
Department of Pharmacology
University of Cambridge
Hills Road
Cambridge
UK

George M. Fanelli, Jr.
Merck Institute for Therapeutic
Research
West Point, PA 19486 USA

D. R. Ferguson
Department of Pharmacology
University of Cambridge
Cambridge
UK

Raymond A. Frizzell
Department of Physiology
University of Pittsburgh
School of Medicine
Pittsburgh, PA 15261 USA

Peter Gund
Merck, Sharp & Dohme Research
Laboratories
Rahway, New Jersey 07065

Sandy I. Helman
Department of Physiology and
Biophysics
University of Illinois
Urbana, IL 61801 USA

S. Hénin
Instituto di Fisologia Generale e di
Chimica Biologica
Universita di Milano
Via Mangiagalli 32
Italy

P. S. James
ARC Institute of Animal
Physiology
Babraham, Cambridge
UK

Leonard B. Kirschner
Department of Zoology
Washington State University
Pullman, WA 99163 USA

B. Lindemann
2nd Department of Physiology
Universität des Saarlandes
6650 Homburg/Saar
West Germany

G. Meyer
Department of Pharmacology
University of Cambridge
Cambridge
UK

Jack Orloff
National Heart and Lung Institute
National Institutes of Health
Bethesda, Maryland 20014

R. Douglas Powers
Department of Biology
Boston College
Chestnut Hill, MA 02167 USA

R. Rick
Physiologishes Institut der
    Universität München
Pettenkoferstrasse 12
D-8000 München 2
West Germany

Ch. Roloff
Physiologisches Institut der
    Universität München
Pettenkoferstrasse 12
D-8000 München 2
West Germany

A. Scriabine
Merck, Sharp & Dohme Research
    Laboratories
West Point, PA 19486 USA

Geoffrey W. G. Sharp
Biochemical Pharmacology Unit
Massachusetts General Hospital
Boston, MA 02114 USA

M. W. Smith
ARC Institute of Animal
    Physiology
Babraham, Cambridge
UK

Robert L. Smith
Merck, Sharp & Dohme Research
    Laboratories
West Point, PA 19486 USA

Larry C. Stoner
Department of Physiology
Upstate Medical Center
SUNY
Syracuse, NY 13210 USA

K. Thurau
Physiologisches Institut der
    Universität München
Pettenkoferstrasse 12
D-8000 München 2
West Germany

Mary Taub
Department of Biology
The University of California, San
    Diego
La Jolla, CA 92093 USA

I. M. Weiner
Department of Pharmacology
Upstate Medical Center
SUNY
Syracuse, NY 13210 USA

S. A. Wilson
Department of Pharmacology
University of Cambridge
Hills Road
Cambridge
UK

Preface

There is something special about a drug when it becomes the subject of an international symposium. This volume includes all those contributions made at a symposium meeting held in Valley Forge, Pennsylvania on April 7, 1978, some eleven years after Cragoe and his colleagues described the synthesis of some N-amidino-3-amino-5-substituted-6-halopyrazinecarboxamides (J Med Chem 10:66, 1967). One of these compounds, the 3,5-diamino-6-chloro derivative was amiloride. As was shown at the Merck Institute for Therapeutic Research, amiloride and many of its analogs possessed modest natriuretic activity and reversed the change in the urinary Na/K ratio in DOCA-treated rats. Subsequently, amiloride proved to be a useful adjunct to diuretic therapy, particularly in view of its potassium-sparing properties. However, these events alone would not account for the substantial interest in this compound at the present time. Of even more importance is the interest generated in amiloride at the basic scientific level which has steadily evolved over the years.

The first inkling that amiloride would be of more than uncommon interest to those working in ion transport came in 1967 when Eigler *et al.*, (Klin Worschr 45:737) showed that amiloride caused a reversible inhibition of sodium transport in frog skin but only when added to the side of the epithelium from which transport was occurring. Numerous studies by many others have confirmed these early discoveries and have also shown similar effects in many other epithelia. As we shall read in this symposium, structures as diverse as the fish gill and the mammalian blastocyst can be included in the list.

Thus, amiloride turns out to be a specific inhibitor of the sodium entry mechanism in the cell membranes of epithelia which, in general, may be described as tight. This property alone has made amiloride a powerful investigative tool for probing a variety of physiological mechanisms, as well as investigating the ion translocation mechanism itself. Unlike most powerful inhibitors of biological processes the actions of amiloride are, generally, readily reversible which adds to its attractiveness as a useful pharmacological tool. Its actions are rather specific and it is probable that its affinity for the sodium entry mechanism is rather high (10^8 M^{-1}) when measured under optimal conditions. Relatively few other effects have been attributed to the drug which are not immediately related to inhibition of sodium entry into cells, but in these instances the concentrations required are very high.

These then are some of the reasons for the continued and increasing interest in this unique compound. Inevitably one is reminded of the stimulus given to research on excitable membranes by the discovery that tetrodotoxin was a selective, reversible and potent inhibitor of the increase in sodium conductance which occurred on excitation. One might suppose that amiloride will be equally important in epithelial studies.

In this symposium we have cast the net wide to cover a variety of interests, from molecular conformation to effects in whole animals. The limitations on time have made it impossible to include other than representatives from the various types of endeavor. Even after the program was completed several notable findings appeared in the literature which are not included among the topics discussed at the symposium. To any who feel left out we apologize, but nevertheless we hope this volume will be a useful reference source for those who work in epithelial transport.

The editors are grateful not only to the Merck Sharp and Dohme Research Laboratories for discovering amiloride and making it available to so many researchers but also to Merck Sharp and Dohme, Division of Merck & Co., Inc. for the support which made this volume a reality.

A. W. Cuthbert
Cambridge
UK

G. M. Fanelli, Jr.
West Point, Pennsylvania
USA

A. Scriabine
West Point, Pennsylvania
USA

October 1978

Structure-Activity Relationships in the Amiloride Series

Edward J. Cragoe, Jr.

Merck Sharp and Dohme Research Laboratories
West Point, Pennsylvania 19486

When the research which ultimately led to the discovery of amiloride began, we were searching for a nonsteroidal saliuretic agent with antikaliuretic properties. One approach to this goal involved screening selected compounds in several animal models in our laboratories. The most rapid screen was an assay in normal rats in which compounds were administered intraperitoneally in doses of 5 and 50 mg/kg. The total urinary Na^+, K^+, Cl^- and urine volume was monitored between 0-5 hr and between 6-24 hr, and the data were scored 0 to 3 in comparison to the standard diuretics shown in Figure 1. The quantitative and qualitative differences among these standards are evident, but they are similar in that they all exhibited kaliuresis.

In the rat screen, in which 20,000 compounds were tested, about a dozen exhibited saliuresis and diuresis with decreased kaliuresis, but compound I proved superior to the others. Thus, this novel pyrazinoyl-guanidine served as a lead for the entire study to be described. Having obtained this prototype which possessed the desired electrolyte excretion profile, the structure was systematically varied in a search for a compound with maximal activity and minimal side-effects.

Due to space limitations and because some of this work has been published elsewhere (see references at the end of this chapter), this paper will be restricted to structure-activity relationships of a few representative compounds selected from among the many which were synthesized. Although the syntheses of the compounds will not be described, I wish to pay tribute to the chemists who were responsible for them: Drs. J.B. Bicking, M.G. Bock, J. Kollonitsch, J.H. Jones, J.W. Mason, K.L. Shepard and R.L. Smith; Misses S.J. deSolms and S.F. Kwong, and

The support, counsel and advice of Drs. K.H. Beyer, R.F. Hirschmann, J.M. Sprague and C.A. Stone are gratefully acknowledged.

1

Drug	0-5 Hrs				6-24 Hrs			
	Na+	K+	Cl⁻	V	Na+	K+	Cl⁻	V
Chlorothiazide	1	1	1	2	0	0	0	0
Hydrochlorothiazide	2	2	2	2	1	1	1	1
Acetazolamide	3	3	1	2	0	0	0	0
Compound I	3	1	2	1	2	0	1	0

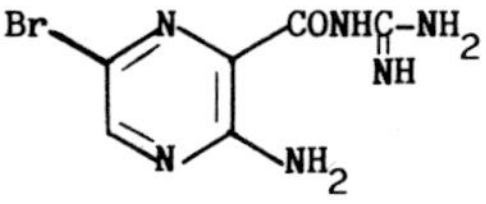

I

Fig. 1.   Normal rat screen.

Dose Producing 50% Reversal of DOCA Na/K Effect, µg/Rat	DOCA Inhibition Score
10	4
10-50	3
51-100	2
101-800	1
800	±
INACTIVE	0

Compounds were evaluated for deoxycorticosterone inhibitory activity. Saline-loaded, adrenalectomized Holtzmann rats weighing 130 $\pm$ 3 g were injected subcutaneously with 12 µg of deoxycorticosterone acetate (DOCA), an amount sufficient to produce a maximal decrease in the urinary ratio of Na/K. The animals were then injected subcutaneously with the test compound and placed in metabolism cages, and 7-hr samples of urine were collected. Analyses of the samples for Na$^+$ and K+ concentrations gave values from which the urinary Na/K ratios could be calculated. The evidence of inhibition of the electrolyte effects of DOCA is a rise in Na/K ratio over that obtained with DOCA alone. The dose of each compound which will produce a 50% reversal of the DOCA effect is listed.

Fig. 2.   ADX rat assay.

Messrs. W. Halczenko, W.J. Holtz, C.M. Robb and O.W. Woltersdorf, Jr. Their research has added an important new chapter to the chemistry of both pyrazines and acylguanidines.

The compounds that were prepared were evaluated in a battery of animal assays. The normal and acetazolamide-loaded rat assays, the dog and chimpanzee assays were designed and conducted by Drs. J.E. Baer, G.M. Fanelli, L.S. Watson, A. Scriabine and Mr. H.F. Russo. The studies in adrenalectomized (ADX) rats were carried out by Dr. M.S. Glitzer and S.L. Steelman. This test was the most precise one for making many of the initial structure-activity judgments. Most of the studies to be presented here were based on ADX rat data. This assay (*Glitzer* and *Steelman*, 1966), which is described in Figure 2, permitted the scoring of compounds from 0 to 4, depending upon the subcutaneous dose required to produce a 50% reversal of 12 μg of deoxycorticosterone. When compound I was tested, about 75 μg was required; therefore, it received a score of 2.

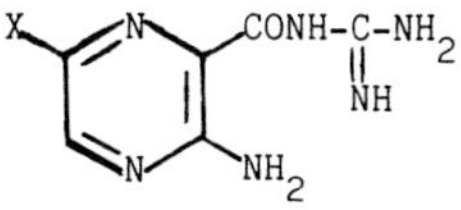

X	ADX RAT SCORE	X	ADX RAT SCORE
(I) Br–	2	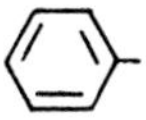 $\bigcirc$–	1
(II) Cl–	3	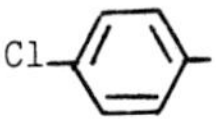 Cl–$\bigcirc$–	±
I–	1	Me_2N–	±
H–	0	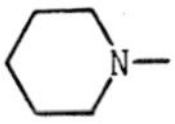 $\bigcirc$N–	±
CF_3–	±	$(CH_3)_2CHNH$–	0
CH_3–	2	$C_6H_5CH_2NH$–	1
C_2H_5–	±	CH_3O–	2
$\triangleright$–	±	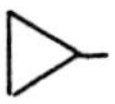 CH_3S–	2
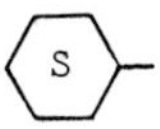 $\langle S \rangle$–	0	CH_3SO_2–	0

Fig. 3. The effect of 6-substituents.

Attention was first focused on the variation of substituents in the 6-position, represented by X in Figure 3. Replacement of the 6-bromo substituent in compound I by chloro (compound II or MK-645) improved the activity, but iodo decreased it. Replacement by H abolished activity and 11 of the other substituents shown had a detrimental effect on activity. Only the 6-methyl, 6-methoxy and 6-methylthio compounds were equal to compound I in potency.

The contribution made by the 5-substituent (Y) is seen in Figure 4. When Y was H, no activity was observed. Of the ten substituents illustrated, only the methoxy and amino (compound III) groups produced an enhancement in activity.

Determination of the optimum combination of 5- and 6-substituents was the next priority (see Fig. 5). Since chloro was the optimal 6-substituent (X), it was held constant while varying the 5-substituent (Y). It was disappointing that none of the combinations shown here was as effective as when Y = H. Surprisingly, when Y = CH_3O a negative effect

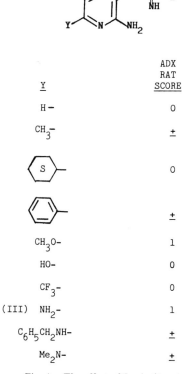

Y	ADX RAT SCORE
H–	0
CH_3–	±
S⟩–	0
⟩–	±
CH_3O–	1
HO–	0
CF_3–	0
(III) NH_2–	1
$C_6H_5CH_2NH$–	±
Me_2N–	±

Fig. 4.   The effect of 5-substituents.

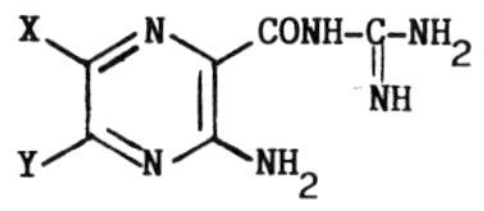

	X	Y	ADX RAT SCORE
(II)	Cl–	H–	3
	Cl–	HO–	$\pm$
	Cl–	CH$_3$O–	$\pm$
	Cl–	C$_2$H$_5$O–	0
	Cl–	HS–	$\pm$
	Cl–	CH$_3$S–	1
	Cl–	Cl–	0

Fig. 5.   The effect of varying both 5- and 6-substituents.

was observed, even though the methoxy group enhanced activity when
X = H (cf. Fig. 4).

Since the 5-amino (Y) group had an enhancing effect on activity
(compound III), this substituent was held constant while various 6-sub-
stituents (X) were introduced (Fig. 6). The 6-chloro compound (IV)
proved to be highly active and received a score of 4, since it produced a

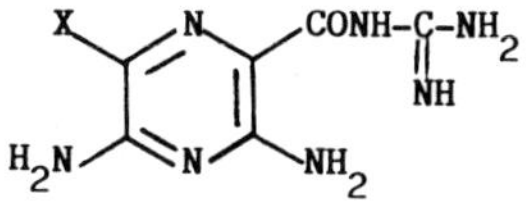

	X	ADX RAT SCORE
(III)	H–	1
(IV)	Cl–	4
	Br–	3
	I–	3

Fig. 6.   The effect of 6-substituents on Compound III.

50% reversal of DOCA effect of 2.5 μg/rat. This compound was first referred to as MK870 and later as amiloride. In this series, the 6-bromo and the 6-iodo analogues were also quite potent.

Figure 7 reveals that when a 5-dimethylamino group is present, introduction of a 6-chloro (compound V) produces a highly active compound (MK685). However, a 6-methyl or 6-phenyl group was not effective. The fact that our most promising compound emanated from this series impelled us to extend the study. Figure 8 shows the four 5-amino-6-substituted (X) compounds recorded in Figure 6, along with five new members of the series. The data provided include the changes during 24 hr in Na^+ and K^+ excretion for normal rats (mean of 3 cages of 3 rats/cage) given 81 mg/kg of each drug as compared to untreated controls. Also, the basicity (pKa) for each compound is recorded. The 6-chloro compound (IV, amiloride) was the most natriuretic and antikaliuretic. Among the new members, the 6-trifluoromethylthio and the 6-fluoro compounds were quite active. The optimal pKa appeared to lie in the 8.7-9.0 range.

A detailed study (Fig. 9) of the four 5-amino-6-halo and the 5-amino-6-H compounds was carried out in normal rats over a three order of magnitude range (0.03 to 30 mg/kg). There was one case of "crossover" in natriuretic activity with varying doses, but the general potency trend was 6-Cl(amiloride) > Br > I > F > H. Within the same experiment (not shown here), the antikaliuretic effects of these compounds were similar.

Figure 10 reveals that variation of the 3-amino substituent on compounds I or II drastically reduced the activity. Substitution of one or

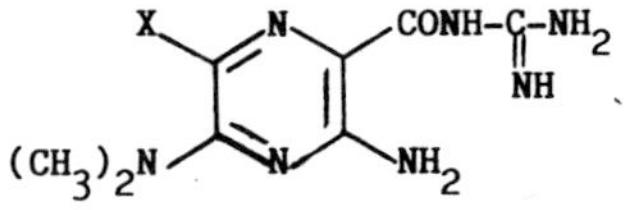

	X	ADX RAT SCORE
	H−	±
(V)	Cl−	4
	CH₃−	1
	C₆H₅−	0

Fig. 7.   The effect of 6-substituents on the 5-dimethyl derivative of III.

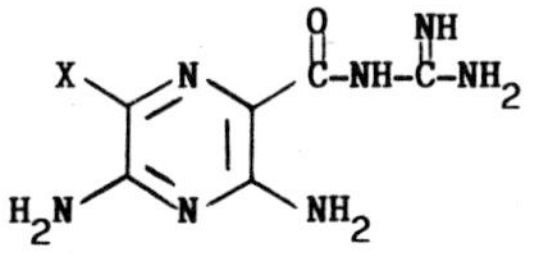

	X	pKa	Difference in electrolyte loss compared to controls in over 24 hours, following a dose of 81 mg/kg orally	
			Na$^+$	K$^+$
	CF$_3$S-	8.20	1.89	-.65
	Br-	8.72	2.55	-.75
(IV)	Cl-	8.80	2.58	-.88
	I-	8.85	1.84	-.39
	CH$_3$S-	8.90		
	F-	9.00	2.24	-.25
(III)	H-	9.30	1.18	-.55
	CN-	10.55	1.41	-.41
	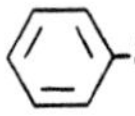 ⬡-S-	-	.37	.08

Fig. 8. The effect of various 6-substituents on Compound III.

both protons of the 3-amino group by methyl slightly reduced the activity. However, substitution by larger groups or replacement of the amino group by other functions virtually abolished activity.

The influence of substituting (R) one of the protons on the 5-amino nitrogen of amiloride (IV) is shown in Figure 11. Activity was optimal only when R was cyclopropylmethyl. When R was a small alkyl group, good activity was observed but large and highly branched groups were not tolerated. Although not shown here, detrimental effects on activity were seen with more complex substituents.

Surprisingly, two substituents on the 5-amino nitrogen (R and R') were better tolerated than one group (Fig. 12). Thus, compounds where R was methyl and R' was ethyl, propyl, or isopropyl were as active as amiloride, and compounds with a combined total of six (aliphatic) carbon atoms (R + R') exhibited very good activity.

Replacement of one of the protons on the terminal nitrogen atom of the guanidino moiety with a variety of substituents (R in Fig. 13) generally produced compounds that were as active as amiloride (IV). This was observed when R was an alkyl, aralkyl, or aryl group. Although not shown here, activity was also maintained when two substituents were placed on one terminal guanidino nitrogen atom or when there was one substituent on each of the two terminal nitrogen atoms. In the latter case, even cyclic analogues were active, i.e., 2-pyrazinamidoimidazolines.

A brief study (Fig. 14) was made involving the replacement of the carbonyl oxygen of the pyrazinoylguanidines by imino (see the encircled portion of compound VI). Note that of the four compounds illustrated, only compound VIA had appreciable activity. This compound, which only scored 1, is the imino analogue of MK685 (V), which had a score of 4.

Figure 15 illustrates the effect of introducing an oxygen atom on the 4-nitrogen atom of the pyrazine ring, thus forming the 4-N-oxides. This produced a dramatic reduction in activity. The last two compounds in the

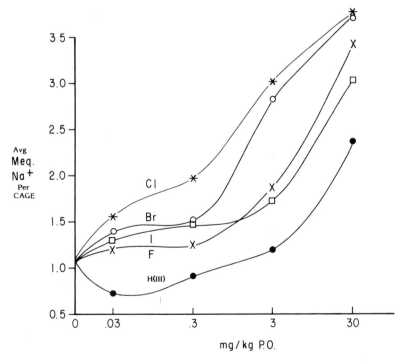

Fig. 9.   6-substituted derivatives of Compound III (0- to 24-hr rat study).

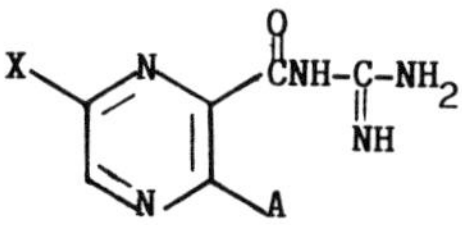

	X	A	SCORE
(I)	Br–	–NH$_2$	2
	Br–	–NHCH$_3$	1
	Br–	–N(CH$_3$)$_2$	1
	Br–	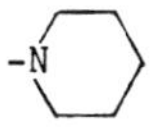 –N⟨piperidine⟩	±
	Br–	–OH	0
	Br–	–SCH$_3$	±
(II)	Cl–	–NH$_2$	3
	Cl–	–NHCH$_2$⟨phenyl⟩ 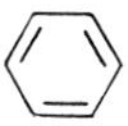	±
	Cl–	–NH–CH$_2$CH$_2$N(CH$_3$)$_2$	±
	Cl–	–OH	±
	Cl–	–OCH$_3$	0
	Cl–	–SH	±

Fig. 10. The effect of modification of the 3-substituent on Compunds I and II.

table, which exhibited only nominal activity, are the 4-N-oxides of
MK645 (II) and amiloride (IV). It will be recalled that II and IV had
scores of 3 and 4, respectively (Figs. 3 and 6).

A most interesting finding (Fig. 16) was that insertion of an NH-
group (see the encircled portion of compound VII) between the carbonyl
carbon and the guanidino moiety of the active pyrazinoylguanidines
produced compounds that were as active as their parents. Thus, the
resulting pyrazinamidoguanidine, such as the 5-H-6-chloro (VIIA) and
the 5-H-6-bromo (VIIB) compounds, were as potent or more potent than
their parents (compounds II and I, respectively). Furthermore, the 5-
amino-6-chloro compound (VIIC) and the 5-dimethylamino-6-chloro
compound (VIID) were also as active as their parents, i.e., amiloride (IV)

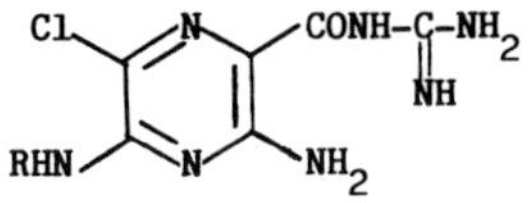

	R	SCORE	R	SCORE
(IV)	H-	4	$t\text{-}C_4H_9-$	±
	CH_3-	3	$C_5H_{11}-$	1
	C_2H_5-	3	$C_3H_7C(CH_3)H-$	1
	C_3H_7-	3	$(C_2H_5)_2CH-$	±
	$i\text{-}C_3H_7-$	3	$C_6H_{13}-$	±
	C_4H_9-	3	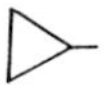 ▷–	3
	$i\text{-}C_4H_9-$	1	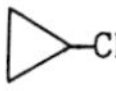 ▷–CH_2-	4
	$sec\text{-}C_4H_9-$	1	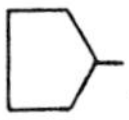 ⬠–	±

Fig. 11.   The effect of one substituent on the 5-amino group of amiloride.

and MK685 (V). Compound VIIC, which was studied in the clinic, is MK875.

It was found that an oxygen atom (see the encircled portion of compound VII in Fig. 17) could be inserted between the carbonyl carbon and the guanidino moiety of amiloride (IV). This structural change produced a dramatic reduction in basicity (over three orders of magnitude below amiloride). However, in comparing the 24-hr electrolyte excretion produced in normal rats over an oral dose range of 3 to 81 mg/kg, it was evident that the natriuretic and antikaliuretic effects were much less than amiloride. Compound VIII was rearranged thermally to give compound IX, in which the oxygen now appears on the terminal guanidino nitrogen atom. This structural change raises the pKa by only one unit, but the natriuretic and antikaliuretic potency was markedly increased.

Replacement of the imino (= NH) group (shown by the symbol Q in compound X of Fig. 18) of the active pyrazinoylguanidines by an oxygen or sulfur atom produced a *qualitative* change in the electrolyte excretion profile. Using the normal rat screen as described in Figure 1, both the pyrazinoylureas (where Q is oxygen, as seen in the first three compounds in the table) and the pyrazinoylthioureas (where Q is sulfur, as seen with compounds IV through VI in the table) exhibited natriuretic properties. However, the potassium-sparing activity exhibited by the pyrazinoyl-guanidines, such as amiloride (IV), had been lost; in fact, compounds XA and XB were frankly kaliuretic.

Some examples of attempts to replace the pyrazine ring with other nuclei are shown in Figure 19. In the first example, the 4-nitrogen atom of compound I was replaced by CH to obtain the corresponding pyridine. Although this compound possessed significant activity, the isomeric compound (second on the list), where the 1-nitrogen atom is replaced by CH, exhibited much weaker activity. The other pyridine analogues, as well as the pyrimidine, thiadiazole, pyrazole, pteridine and benzene analogues, had little or no activity. Improper nuclear substitution may have contributed to the negative results.

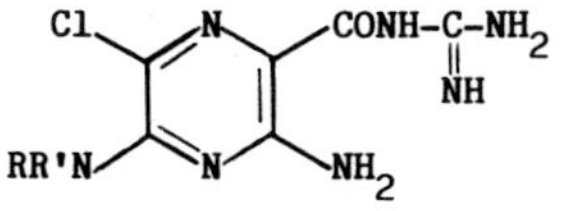

	R	R'	SCORE
(V)	CH_3-	CH_3-	4
	C_2H_5-	C_2H_5-	3
	CH_3-	C_2H_5-	4
	CH_3-	C_3H_7-	4
	CH_3-	$i-C_3H_7-$	4
	CH_3-	C_4H_9-	3
	C_2H_5-	C_3H_7-	3
	C_2H_5-	C_4H_9-	3
	C_3H_7-	C_4H_9-	1
	$-(CH_2)_4-$		1
	CH_3-	CH_3O-	2
	CH_3-	NH_2-	1

Fig. 12.   The effect of two substituents on the 5-amino group of amiloride.

Figure 20 illustrates the basicity (pKa) and lipophilic-hydrophilic character (measured as the distribution ratio between chloroform and pH 7.4 buffer) of a number of the more active compounds which were described earlier in both the pyrazinoylguanidine and the pyrazinamidoguanidine series. It can be seen that the most potent compounds, i.e., amiloride (II) and MK875 (VIIA), have pKa values in the 8.6 to 9.0 range and are distributed almost completely in the aqueous phase.

In Figure 21 the activity of amiloride is compared with that of spironolactone and triamterene. First, the dose of each drug required in the ADX assay to produce a 50% inhibition of 12 μg of DOCA is shown. In this assay, amiloride was 160 times more potent than spironolactone and 32 times more potent than triamterene. A comparison of the recommended clinical doses, allegedly required to produce equivalent clinical

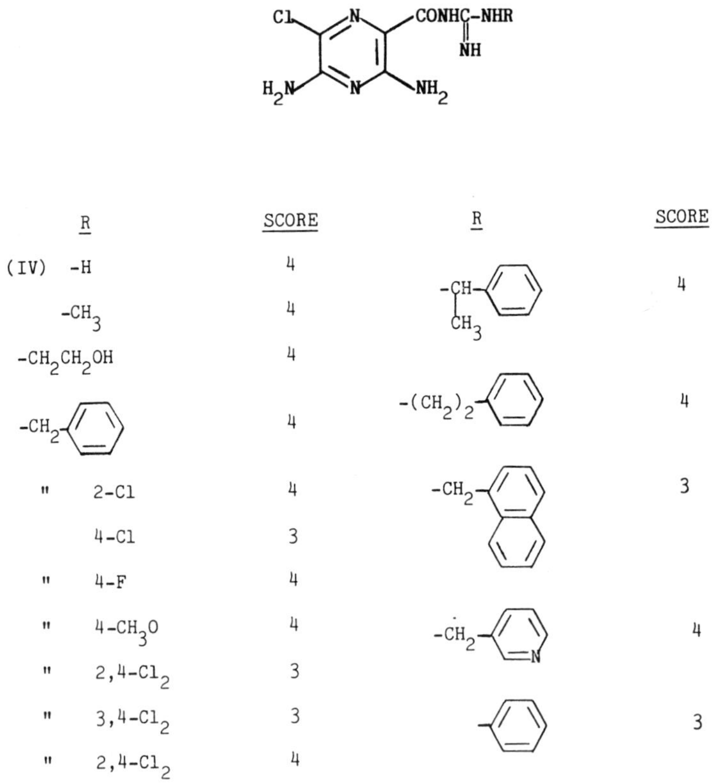

R	SCORE	R	SCORE
(IV) -H	4	-CH- with CH₃ and phenyl (-$\overset{|}{\underset{CH_3}{CH}}$-C₆H₅)	4
-CH₃	4		
-CH₂CH₂OH	4		
-CH₂-phenyl	4	-(CH₂)₂-phenyl	4
" 2-Cl	4	-CH₂-naphthyl	3
4-Cl	3		
" 4-F	4		
" 4-CH₃O	4	-CH₂-pyridyl	4
" 2,4-Cl₂	3		
" 3,4-Cl₂	3		
" 2,4-Cl₂	4	phenyl	3

Fig. 13.   The effect of substituting the terminal guanidino nitrogen of amiloride.

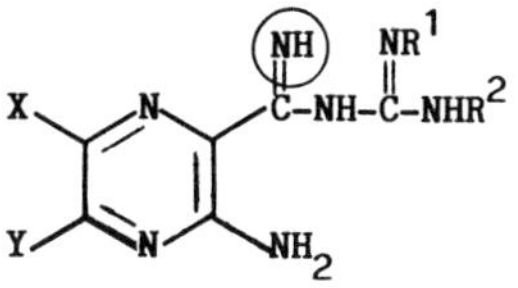

VI

X	Y	R^1	R^2
H-	H-	H-	H-
Cl-	H-	-(CH$_2$)$_2$-	
Cl-	Cl-	-(CH$_2$)$_2$-	
VIA Cl-	Me$_2$N-	H-	H-

Fig. 14. The effect of replacing the carbonyl oxygen of MK685.

effects, is given. Using this criterion, amiloride was 5 to 20 times more potent than spironolactone and 20 times more so than triamterene.

It might be thought that the pyrazinoylguanidines (Fig. 22, compound IV) are obvious "ring-opened" or seco analogues of the diuretic pteridines, such as "chloramterene" (XIA where X is chloro) and triamterene (where X is phenyl). However, there is little to support this

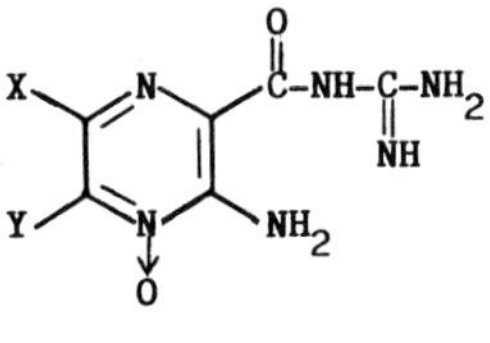

X	Y	ADX RAT SCORE
H-	H-	1
Cl-	H-	±
Cl-	NH$_2$-	±

Fig. 15. The effect of forming the 4-N-oxide of amiloride.

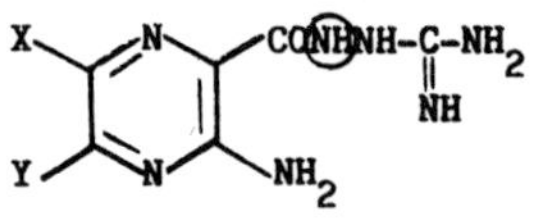

VII

	X	Y	SCORE
	H–	H–	±
VIIA	Cl–	H–	3
(4-0)	Cl–	H–	±
VIIB	Br–	H–	3
	I–	H–	1
	H–	CF_3^-	±
VIIC	Cl–	NH_2^-	4
	Cl–	$(CH_3)_2CHNH–$	3
	Cl–	AllylNH–	2
VIID	Cl–	$Me_2N–$	4

Fig. 16.   The effect of inserting an NH group between the carbonyl and guanidino moiety of amiloride.

notion. Hydrolysis of XIA or XIB to the corresponding 4-hydroxy-pteridine (XII) produced a dramatic reduction in activity. Further, hydrolysis to the pyrazinoylureas (X) was not beneficial since these compounds are only weakly natriuretic and are frankly kaliuretic.

Ammonolysis of XI to VI produced compounds with very weak activity. The selective hydrolysis required to convert VI to IV has never been observed *in vivo;* in fact, what is observed in the laboratory is the reverse reaction, i.e., the facile cyclization of compounds of type VI to the corresponding pteridines (XI). Of course, ammonolysis of XII or X (to IV) is a chemical process without precedent in the literature and it has not been observed in our laboratories. Finally, amiloride is much more basic (pKa 8.7) than triamterene (6.2); therefore, under physiological conditions, amiloride is expected to exist largely in the protonated form, while triamterene should exist mainly as the free base.

	pKa
(VIII)	4.50
(IX)	5.48
AMILORIDE (IV)	8.7

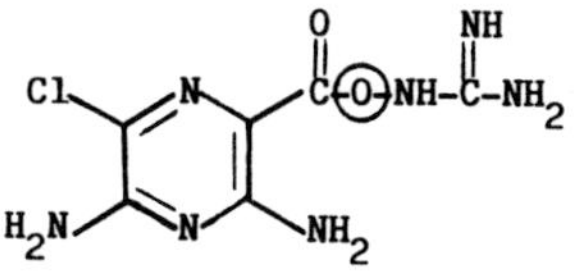

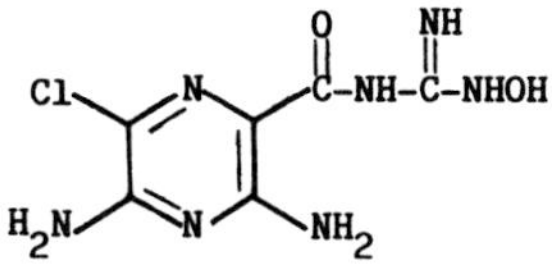

ORAL DOSE (mg/kg/rat)   mEq. x 100/cage/24 hours

ORAL DOSE	Na$^+$			K$^+$		
	VIII	IX	IV	VIII	IX	IV
0	.80	.80	.80	1.07	1.07	1.07
3	.92	2.47	3.06	1.11	1.10	1.78
9	.97	3.08	3.78	1.08	.90	1.66
27	1.89	3.47	4.57	.96	.70	1.53
81	2.29	3.88	4.60	.72	.63	.50

Fig. 17. The effect of inserting an oxygen atom between the carbonyl and guanidino moiety of amiloride.

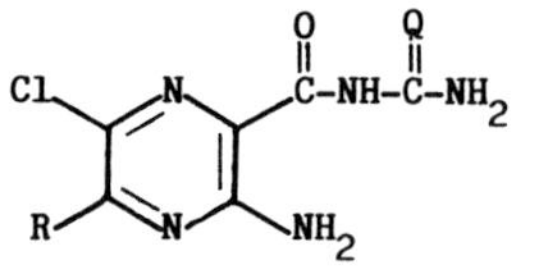

X

R	Q	Mg/Kg Dose	NORMAL RAT SCREENING SCORE Na^i	K$^+$
H−	O	50	2	1
(CH$_3$)$_2$N−	O	50	1	1
(XA) NH$_2$−	O	50	2	2
H−	S	50	1	2
C$_2$H$_5$NH−	S	50	0	1
(XB) NH$_2$−	S	50	2	1
(IV) NH$_2$−	NH	5	3	0 (−K)

Fig. 18.   The effect of replacing the guanidino NH of amiloride by oxygen or sulfur.

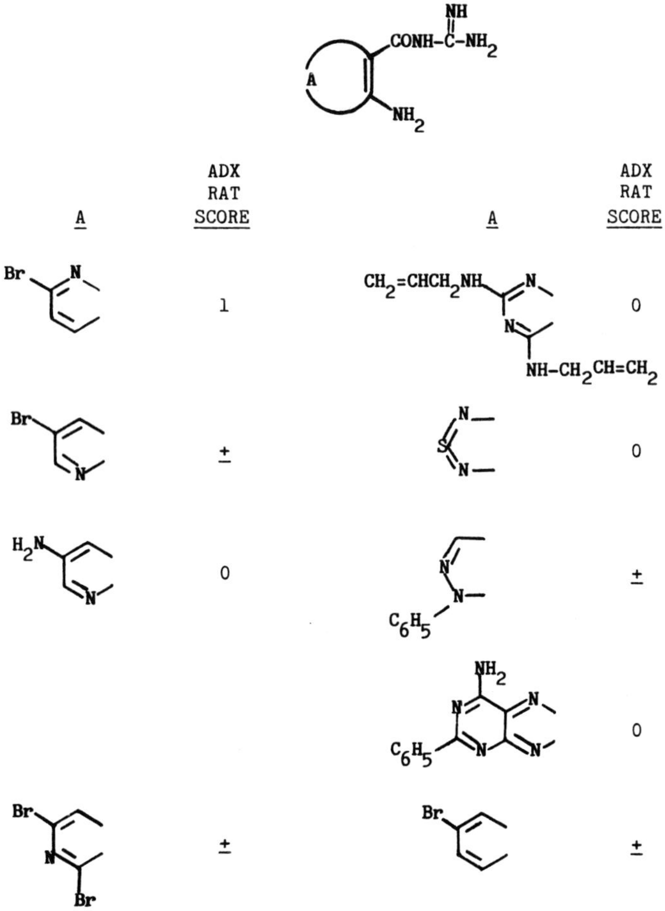

Fig. 19. The effect of replacing the pyrazine ring.

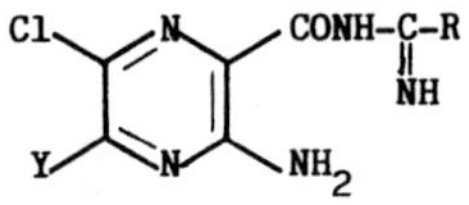

Y	R	pKa	CHCl$_3$/7.4 BUFFER
H-	-NH$_2$	7.03	0.02
(CH$_3$)$_2$N-	-NH$_2$	8.76	0.06
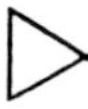 ▷-CH$_2$NH-	-NH$_2$	8.90	0.06
(IV) NH$_2$-	-NH$_2$	8.67	0.01
NH$_2$-	-NHCH$_2$CH$_2$OH	8.68	0.02
NH$_2$-	-NHCH$_2$C$_6$H$_5$	8.10	2.01
(CH$_3$)$_2$CHNH	-N(CH$_3$)$_2$	7.85	∞
NH$_2$-	-NHOH	5.48	0.17

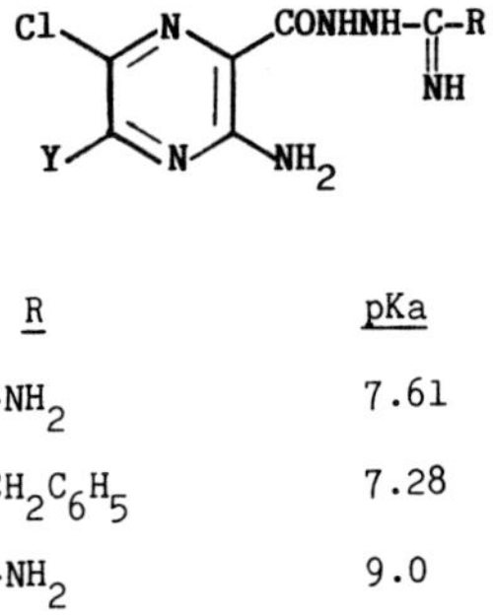

Y	R	pKa	CHCl$_3$/7.4 BUFFER
H-	-NH$_2$	7.61	0.01
H-	-NHCH$_2$C$_6$H$_5$	7.28	1.22
VIIA NH$_2$-	-NH$_2$	9.0	0.01

Fig. 20.   The effect of structure on basicity and hydrophilicity.

COMPOUND	ADX RAT ASSAY (μg Required for 50% Inhib. of DOCA)	CLINICAL DOSE (mg)
Amiloride	2.5	5
Spironolactone	400	25-100
Triamterene	80	100

Fig. 21.

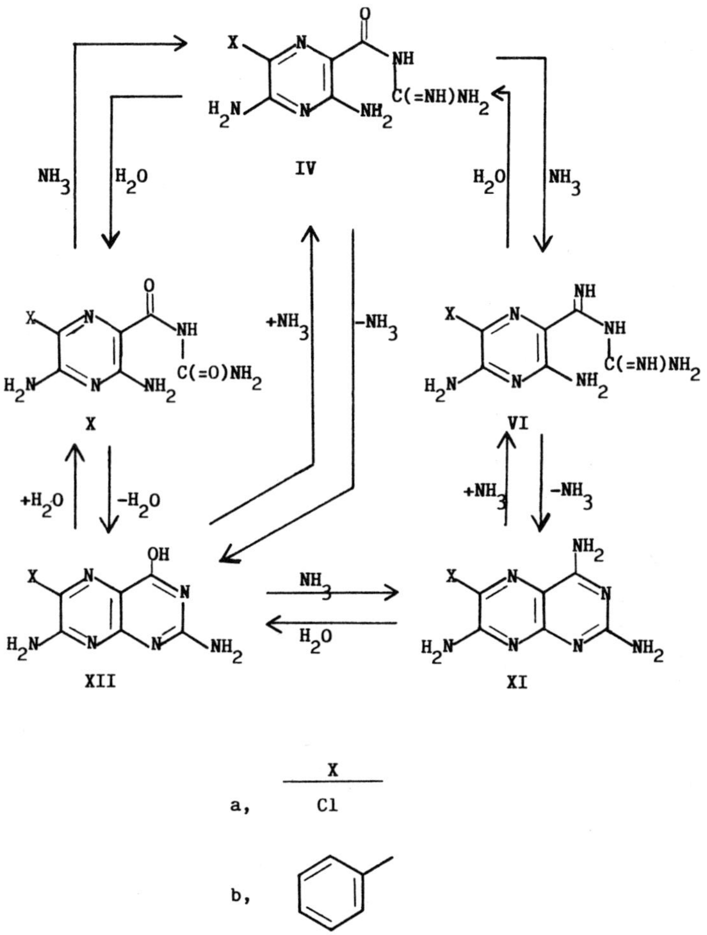

Fig. 22.   Comparisons of pyrazinoylguanidines with the corresponding pteridines.

REFERENCES

Bicking, J.B., Mason, J.W., Woltersdorf, O.W., Jr., Jones, J.H., Kwong, S.F.,
   Robb, C.M., and Cragoe, E.J., Jr.   1965.   Pyrazine diuretics. I. N-amidino-
   3-amino-6-halopyrazinecarboxamides. J Med Chem 8:638–642
Bicking, J.B., Robb, C.M., Kwong, S.F., and Cragoe, E.J., Jr.   1967.   Pyrazine
   diuretics. III. 5- and 6-alkyl, -cycloalkyl and -aryl derivatives of N-amidino-3-
   aminopyrazinecarboxamides. J Med Chem 10:598–602
Cragoe, E.J., Jr., Woltersdorf, O.W., Jr., Bicking, J.B., Kwong, S.F., and Jones,
   J.H.   1967.   Pyrazine diuretics. II. N-amidino-3-amino-5-substituted 6-
   halopyrazines. J Med Chem 10:66–75
Cragoe, E.J., Jr., Schultz, E.M., Schneeberg, J.D., Stokker, G.E., Woltersdorf,
   O.W., Jr., Fanelli, G.M., Jr., and Watson, L. S.   1975.   (1-oxo-2-substituted-

5-indanyloxy)acetic acids, a new class of potent renal agents possessing both uricosuric and saluretic activity. A reexamination of the role of sulfhydryl binding in the mode of action of acylphenoxyacetic acid saluretics. J Med Chem 18:225–228

Glitzer, M.S., and Steelman, S.L.   1966.   N-amidino-3,5-diamino-6-chloro-pyrazinecarboxamide. A potent diuretic in the carboxamide series which antagonizes the renal actions of aldosterone. Nature (Lond) 212:191–193

Jones, J.H., Bicking, J.B., and Cragoe, E.J., Jr.   1967.   Pyrazine diuretics. IV. N-Amidino-3-amino-6-Substituted Pyrazinecarboxamides. J Med Chem 10:899–903

Jones, J.H., and Cragoe, E.J., Jr.   1968.   Pyrazine diuretics. V. N-amidino-3-amino-pyrazinecarboxamides and analogous 2,4-diaminopteridines. J Med Chem 11:322–325

Jones, J.H., Holtz, W.J., and Cragoe, E.J., Jr.   1969.   Pyrazine diuretics. VII. N-amidino-3-substituted pyrazinecarboxamides. J Med Chem 12:285–287

Jones, J.H., and Cragoe, E.J., Jr.   1970.   Pyrazine diuretics. VIII. N-amidino-3-aminopyrazinecarboxamide 4-oxides. J Med Chem 13:987–991

Shepard, K.L., Mason, J.W., Woltersdorf, O.W., Jr., Jones, J. H., and Cragoe, E.J., Jr.   1969.   Pyrazine diuretics. VI. (Pyrazinecarboxamido)guanidines. J Med Chem 12:280–285

Shepard, K.L., Halczenko, W., and Cragoe, E.J., Jr.   1969.   3,5-diamino-6-chloropyrazinecarboxylic acid "active esters" and their reactions (1). Tetrahedron Lett 54:4757–4760

Shepard, K.L., Halczenko, W., and Cragoe, E.J., Jr.   1976.   Activated esters of substituted pyrazinecarboxylic acids (1). J Hetero Chem 13:1219–1224

Amiloride and Epithelial Sodium Transport
Edited by A.W. Cuthbert, G.M. Fanelli, Jr. and A. Scriabine

Studies on the Tautomerism and Conformation of Amiloride

Robert L. Smith*, David W. Cochran*, Edward J. Cragoe, Jr.*
and Peter Gund**

*Merck Sharp and Dohme Research Laboratories
West Point, Pennsylvania 19486
**Merck Sharp and Dohme Research Laboratories
Rahway, New Jersey 07065

As noted in the preceding paper in this volume (*Cragoe*, Structure-Activity Relationships in the Amiloride Series), the discovery by *Bicking et al.* (1965) that certain acylguanidines such as compound 1 display natriuretic activity while repressing kaliuresis in experimental animals led to an extensive synthetic program based on this novel class of structures. This program culminated with the development (*Glitzer* and *Steelman*, 1966) of amiloride (2), which subsequently was shown to be a clinically effective potassium-sparing diuretic agent when used either alone (*Schapel*, *Edwards*, and *Robinson*, 1975) or in combination with hydrochlorothiazide, i.e., as Moduretic (*Burge* and *Montuschi*, 1976). Furthermore, in recent years amiloride has emerged as a unique investigational tool for probing sodium translocation mechanisms in biological systems, particularly in amphibian skin preparations (*Cuthbert*, 1976; *Benos et al.*, 1976). Although the pharmacological basis accounting for amiloride's renotropic properties appears to be well established (*Baer* and *Beyer*, 1972; *Stoner*, *Burg*, and *Orloff*, 1974), elucidation of its mechanism of action at the molecular level is yet to be achieved. To do

The authors wish to thank Mr. Len Olen for assistance with the CNDO/2 calculations, Mr. O.W. Woltersdorf for synthesis of ^{13}C-labeled amiloride, Ms. S.J. deSolms for preparation of model compound 4 and Dr. W.C. Randall and his staff for elemental analyses and pKa determinations. We are indebted to Mr. J. Hirshfield and Drs. J. Springer and K. Hoogsteen for the X-ray crystallographic analysis of amiloride. Gratitude is expressed to Profs. John Baldeschwieler and Barry Trost and to our colleagues, Drs. Byron Arison, Mark Bock and Alvin Willard, for constructive criticism and useful suggestions on various aspects of this investigation and to Prof. J.D. Roberts for allowing one of us (D. W. C.) to use his ^{15}N NMR facilities. We are deeply indebted to Dr. Ralph Hirschmann for helpful discussions and encouragement throughout the course of these studies.

so will necessitate both the determination of the active *in vivo* conformation(s) of amiloride and the isolation and structural characterization of the appropriate renal receptor(s) or binding site(s). In principle, attainment of these objectives will contribute to a better understanding of the dynamic structural properties of acylguanidines and, concomitantly, faciliate the rational design of future diuretic agents with improved therapeutic attributes.

As an approach toward achieving these goals, the structural dynamics of amiloride and other members of the pyrazinoylguanidine series were investigated in our laboratories using both empirical (NMR,

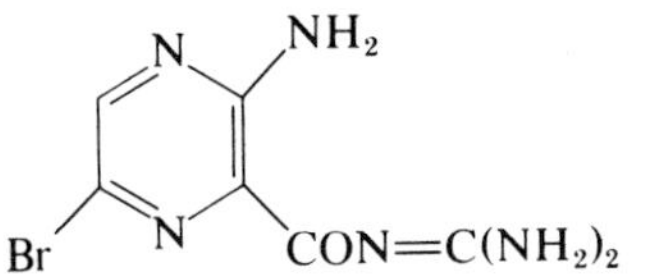

1

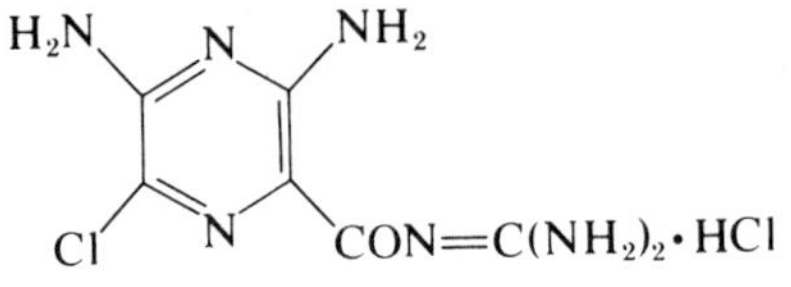

2

IR) and theoretical (CNDO/2) techniques, the latter serving to guide the experimental approach. The results of this investigation provided a basis for effecting a subsequent dynamic structure-activity analysis (*Ganellin*, 1977) of the amiloride series. Herein, we wish to present the main points of our recently completed studies on the tautomerism and conformation of amiloride, the details of which are described elsewhere (*Smith et al.*, in press).

GROUND-STATE TAUTOMER FORM

The pKa (8.7) of amiloride implies that the drug exists predominantly as a cation (i.e., as an acylguanidinium ion) in the physiologic pH range, particularly in renal tubular fluid. However, in view of the structural complexity of amiloride, its remarkable chemical stability (*in vitro* and *in vivo*) in aqueous milieu and the paucity of information currently available on the dynamic structural properties of acylguanidines, it was deemed essential that both the protonated and free-base drug forms be rigorously studied in this investigation.

Three likely (i.e., low-energy) tautomeric forms, the acylamino 3a, acylimino 3b and isoimino 3c types, are available to acylguanidines devoid of nitrogen substituents. Each of these tautomeric forms can be interconverted formally via 1,3- and 1,5-prototropic shifts as illustrated below. Likewise, the existence and interconversion of their conjugate acids (i.e., $RCONHC(=N^+H_2)NH_2$, etc.) are possible.

$$\overset{\overset{\displaystyle O}{\|}}{R}C\overset{\overset{\displaystyle NH_2}{|}}{N}=CNH_2$$

3b

1,3-H
Shift

1,5-H
Shift

(1) $$R\overset{\overset{\displaystyle O}{\|}}{C}NH\overset{\overset{\displaystyle NH}{\|}}{C}NH_2$$

3a

1,3-H
Shift

$$R\overset{\overset{\displaystyle OH}{|}}{C}=N\overset{\overset{\displaystyle NH}{\|}}{C}NH_2$$

3c

R = alkyl, aryl

Several lines of experimental and theoretical evidence led to the conclusion that, in those solvents studied, primarily dimethyl sulfoxide and dimethyl sulfoxide-methanol, amiloride exists predominantly in the acylamino tautomer form, $RCONHC(=N^+H_2)NH_2$, whereas the free base of the drug prefers to assume the acylimino tautomer form, $RCON=C(NH_2)_2$, where R is the 3,5-diamino-6-chloropyrazinyl moiety (Equation 1). First, the striking similarities in ^{13}C chemical shifts and $\Delta\delta$ values (magnitude and direction of shift) upon protonation observed for the free base of amiloride, as well as its terminally substituted tetramethyl derivative [$RCON=C(NR'_2)_2$ where $R'=CH_3$] and creatinine, suggested that these structures exist in a common tautomeric form. The N-terminally substituted derivative of amiloride, by virtue of substituent-imposed geometrical constraints, must assume the acylimino tautomer form. This tautomer form was previously assigned to creatinine based on UV and NMR spectral evidence (*Matsumoto* and *Rappoport*, 1968; *Stearns* and *Rappoport*, 1977). Further support for these tautomer assignments emerged from the ^{15}N NMR spectra recorded for amiloride and its free-base form. The spin-coupled ^{15}N NMR spectrum of amiloride displayed six peaks: a triplet due to the terminal NH_2 groups (i.e., the $-C(=N^+H_2)NH_2$ fragment), a doublet resulting from the amide-type nitrogen atom ($RCONH-$) and four peaks arising from the nitrogen atoms incorporated in (N-1, N-4) and appended to (3-NH_2, 5-NH_2) the pyrazine ring. Likewise, the neutral drug form exhibited a six-signal spin-coupled ^{15}N NMR spectrum. However, in addition to notable chemical shift differences reflecting the absence of a positive charge, this spectrum differed from that of amiloride in that it contained a singlet arising from the acylimino nitrogen atom [$RCON=C(NH_2)_2$]. Finally, the presence of a broad singlet at δ 10 (RCON*H*—) in the ^{1}H NMR spectrum of amiloride and, conversely, the absence of such a signal in the ^{1}H NMR spectrum of the free-base form, served to corroborate these tautomer assignments.

GROUND-STATE CONFORMATION

Having established the preferred ground-state tautomer forms for amiloride and its free base, we next determined their respective ground-state conformations through the concomitant use of the CNDO/2 formalism and NMR experimental methods. As shown in Figure 1, these studies led to the conclusion that the free-base form of amiloride most likely exists in the ground state as either conformer A1 and/or conformer A4. Although the evidence in hand did not allow a choice to be made between these two likely conformations, interestingly, their protonation leads to a single ground-state structure (F1) for amiloride.

As indicated in Figure 1, conformers A1, A4 and F1 are characterized by several common structural features. The designated intramolecular hydrogen bonds, calculated by the CNDO/2 method to have strengths ranging from approximately 4.7 to 6.1 kcal/mole, serve to impart molecular planarity to each of these conformers. The imparted

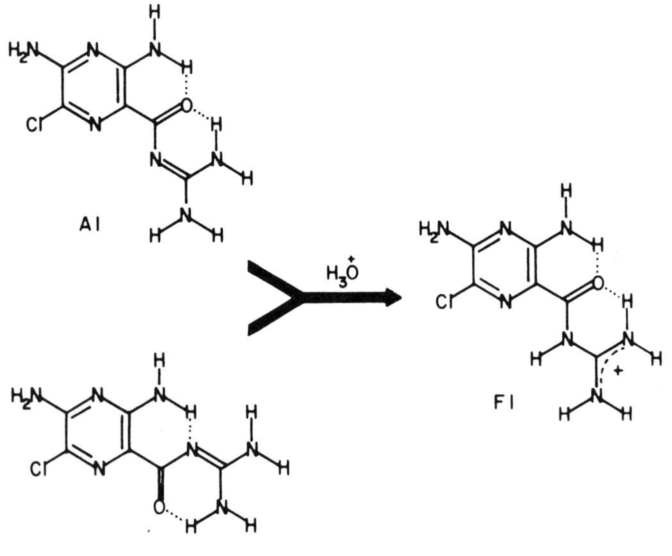

Fig. 1.   Ground-state conformations of amiloride (F1) and its free-base form (A1, A4).

planarity, in turn, is conducive to maximal conjugative interaction between the pyrazinecarbonyl and guanidine moieties and, thereby, substantially contributes to the known chemical stability of these structures. The possible importance of the intramolecular bond between the 3-NH_2 group and the carbonyl oxygen atom to biological activity is revealed by the data tabulated in Figure 10 of the preceding paper in this volume (*Cragoe*, Structure-Activity Relationships in the Amiloride Series). The latter strongly suggests that introduction of substituents in the 3-position which are either incapable of hydrogen bond donation or are relatively poor hydrogen bond donors is detrimental to biological activity. The rapid interconversion of their terminal NH_2 groups, a dynamic structural feature common to both amiloride and its free-base form, will be discussed in the next section.

The different locales indicated for the $C{=}N$, the major dissimilarity between conformers A1 (and A4) and F1, stems from the fact that whereas structures A1 and A4 are neutral species with the $C{=}N$ directed toward the internal nitrogen atom (i.e., $RCON{=}C(NH_2)_2$), conformer F1 is a cationic structure in which the positive charge is delocalized on the terminal amidinium fragment (i.e., $RCONHC({=}NH_2)NH_2$). Indeed, the experimentally observed upfield shift in the carbonyl group ^{13}C resonance position, i.e., from a position expected for a highly shielded ketone to a position more characteristic of a typical amide, which accompanies the conversion (via protonation) of A1 and/or A4 to F1 is consistent with these conformational assignments. Finally, it should be noted that the solid-state structure of amiloride (crystals deposited from dimethyl sulfoxide), determined by the single crystal X-ray crystallographic technique (*Hirshfield, Springer*, and *Hoogsteen*, unpublished results) after the presentation of this paper, is in complete accord with ground-state conformation F1.

DYNAMIC CONFORMATION

Equivalence of the terminal amino groups was observed in the ^{15}N NMR spectra recorded for amiloride and its free-base form (*vide supra*). Likewise, in each terminally substituted amiloride derivative studied, either as the neutral or the protonated species, the terminal amino groups and their N-substituents displayed ^{1}H, ^{13}C and ^{15}N NMR equivalence. These observations implied that the guanidino and, when protonated, guanidinium NH_2 groups, as well as their substituents (when N-substituted), were interconverting (i.e., undergoing an exchange of their relative spatial positions) rapidly on the NMR time scale. Hence, our investigation was next directed toward elucidating the mechanism(s) by which this dynamic equilibration occurs.

A priori, at least six distinct pathways can be envisioned for equilibrating the terminal NH_2 groups in the free-base form of amiloride. The first pathway (Path A in Fig. 2) which was considered involves the processes of tautomerism and rotation. Conformer A1 initially undergoes a 1,3-prototropic shift to afford conformer B3 which, upon subsequent rotation about the newly generated C—N bond, leads to conformer B2. A subsequent 1,3-prototropic shift provides conformer A1' and, thereby, completes this interconversion pathway. A second pathway (Path B in Fig. 3) is similar to Path A but involves an initial intramolecular 1,5-prototropic shift and terminates via an intermolecular tautomerism process. The observed N—H coupling (i.e., a single triplet for the terminal NH_2 groups) in both amiloride and its free-base form is inconsistent with any mechanism involving intermolecular proton exchange and, therefore, served to exclude Paths A and B as major equilibration pathways in this instance.

A third possible equilibration mechanism, simple rotation about the C=N linkage, is depicted by Path C in Figure 4. The fourth mechanism considered proceeds by way of processes involving both rotation and

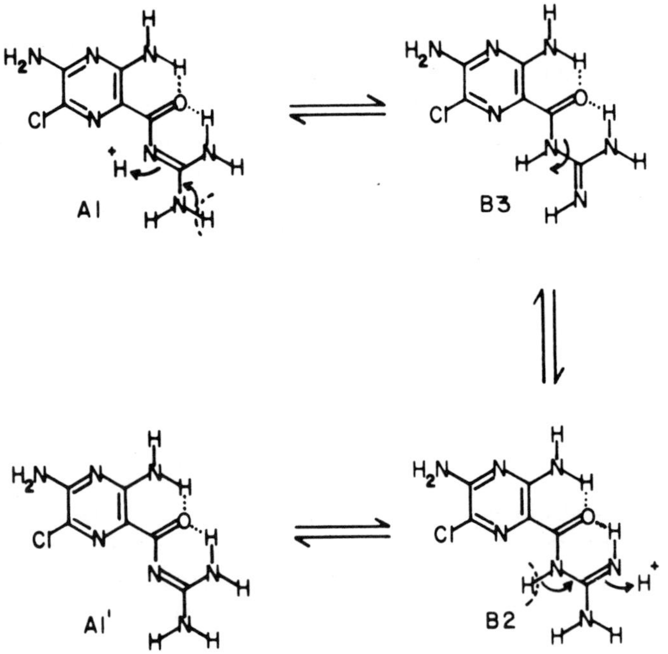

Fig. 2.   Path A: Equilibration via tautomerism (1,3-H shift) and rotation.

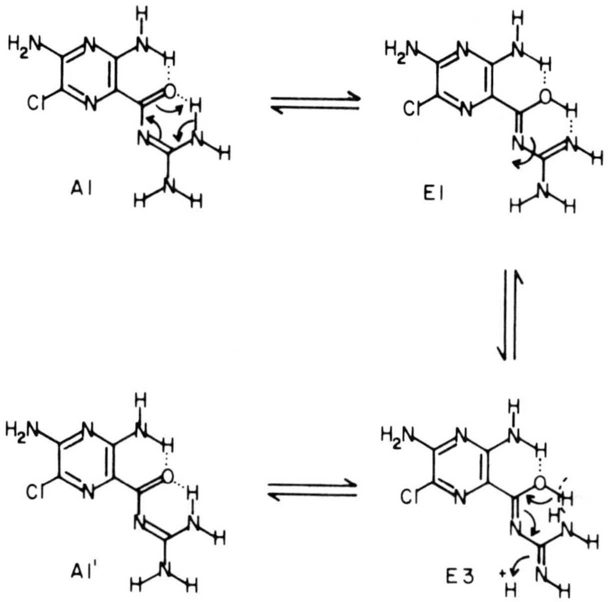

Fig. 3.   Path B: Equilibration via tautomerism (1,5-H shift) and rotation.

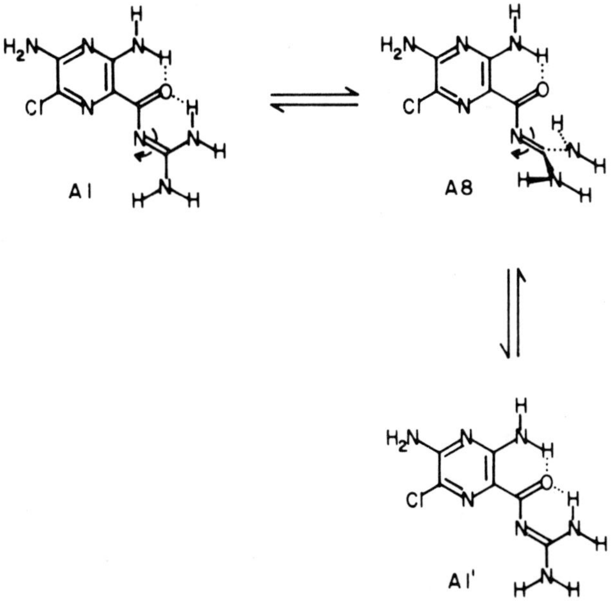

Fig. 4.   Path C: Equilibration via simple rotation.

inversion as shown by Path D in Figure 5. In this pathway, conformer A1 first undergoes rotation about the designated C—N bond to afford conformer A6 which, upon inversion of the amide nitrogen, gives rise to conformer A6' by way of conformer E4 which bears an sp-hybridized, linear amide nitrogen. Rotation about the designated C—N bond completes this equilibration process. Path E, presented in Figure 6, also proceeds by way of inversion and rotation but in a sequence reversed from that in Path D.

The sixth and last mechanistic pathway considered in our studies, Path F in Figure 7, was calculated to have the lowest energy transition state, A23, the latter representing in effect an "internally solvated" species. The key dynamic event in Path F is the interconversion of conformers A6 and A6' via the designated "synchronized" rotations which

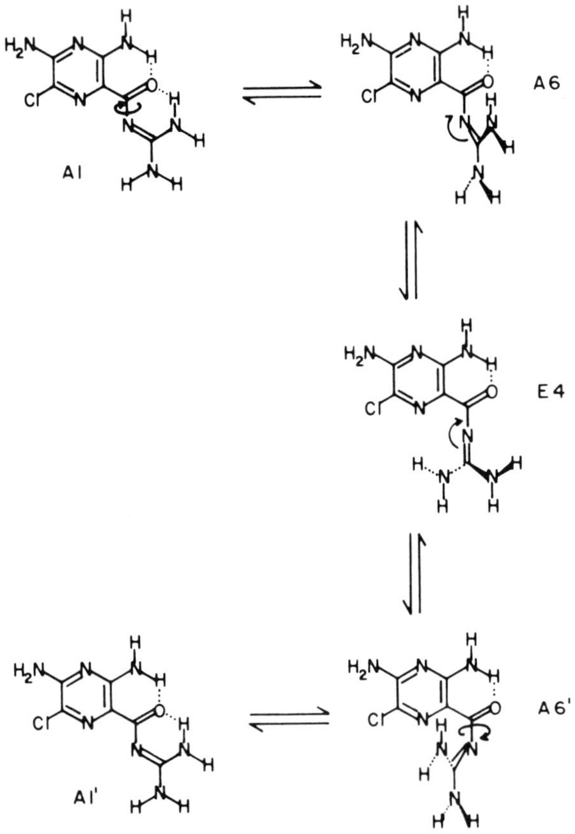

Fig. 5.   Path D: Equilibration via rotation and inversion.

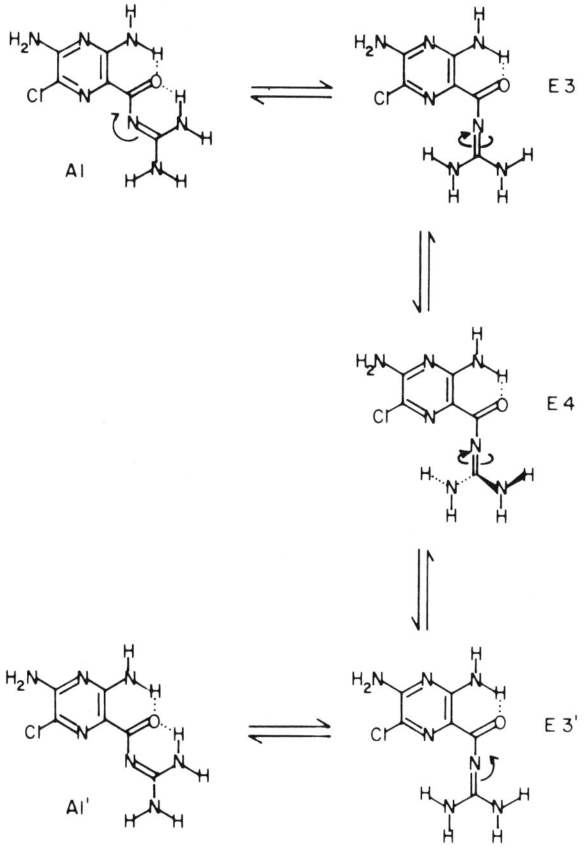

Fig. 6.   Path E: Equilibration via inversion and rotation.

pass through A23. In view of recent X-ray crystallographic studies which suggest that molecules in biological active sites may well be present as desolvated entities, particularly in hydrophobic pockets, it was deemed important to explore Path F in detail. If this pathway represented the "true" equilibration mechanism as was predicted by the CNDO/2 formalism, removal of the stabilizing nonbonding interaction between the pyrazine 1-position and the guanidine carbon present in A23, e.g., by isosteric replacement of nitrogen (i.e., N-1) with carbon, should substantially elevate the energy of the synchronized rotation mechanism. This hypothesis was tested by calculating the free energy of activation, $\Delta G\ddagger$, at the experimentally determined (dynamic ^{13}C NMR technique) coalescence temperature, T_c, for model compound 4 and amiloride derivative 5 and its hydrochloride salt.

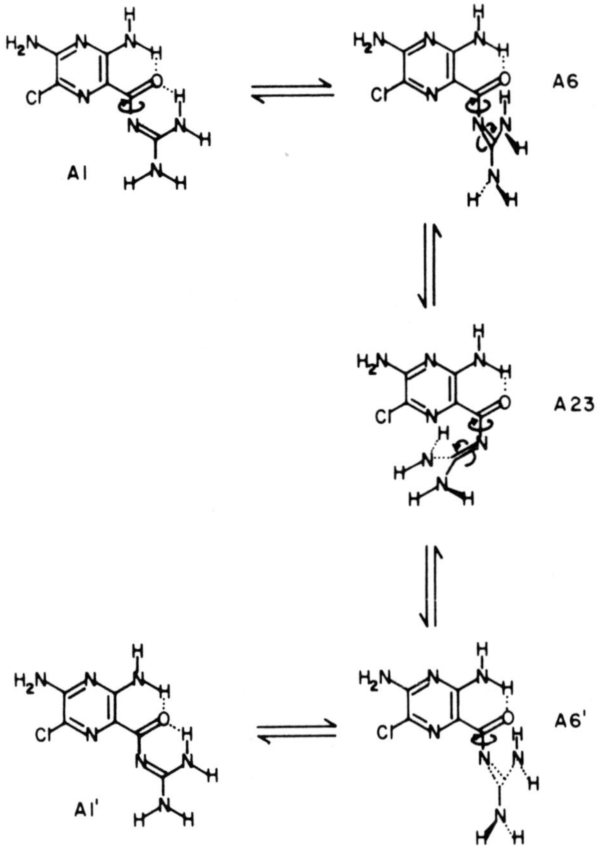

Fig. 7.   Path F: Equilibration via synchronized rotation.

The $\Delta G\ddagger$ values (*ca.* 14.7 kcal/mole) calculated for compounds 4, 5 and 5.HCl were identical (within experimental error) and, therefore, suggested that Path F is not operant for these structures, at least under the experimental conditions studied. Accordingly, our data led us to conclude that the free base of amiloride probably undergoes dynamic equilibration by either the simple rotation or rotation plus inversion pathways, or both; a choice between these mechanisms could not be made. On the other hand, since the inversion mechanism is precluded for tetravalent nitrogen, the only dynamic pathway open to amiloride is simple rotation (Path C).

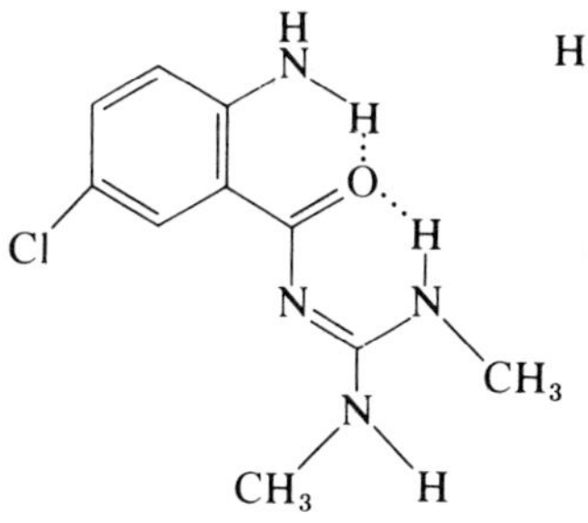

4 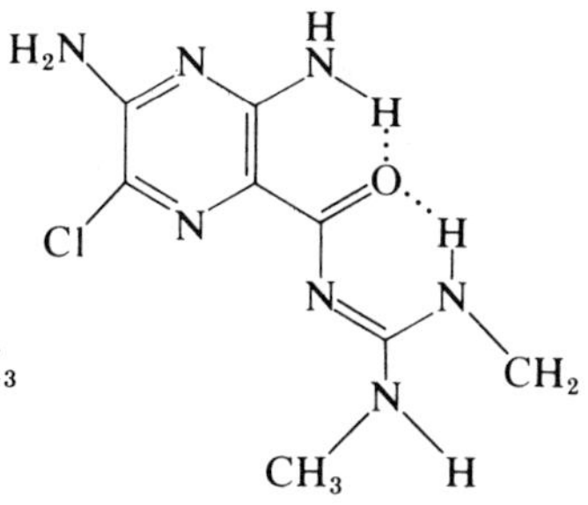   5

SUMMARY AND CONCLUSIONS

In summary, these studies indicate that amiloride exists predominately in the ground state in planar conformation F1. The observed intramolecular hydrogen bonding between the salient functional groups and the maximum π overlap between the pyrazinoyl and guanidinium moieties attendant with their coplanar spatial orientation no doubt account, at least in part, for the favorable energetics ascribed to planar conformer F1. These conformational features serve to explain the known chemical stability of amiloride in aqueous milieu. The dynamic NMR results strongly suggest that amiloride achieves the observed rapid interconversion of its terminal NH_2 groups via a process involving simple rotation about the C—N bond in the guanidinium moiety. However, the possibility remains that the synchronized rotation mechanism may represent a competing dynamic equilibration pathway, particularly in nonpolar media, *in vacuo* or within a biological active site.

(2)

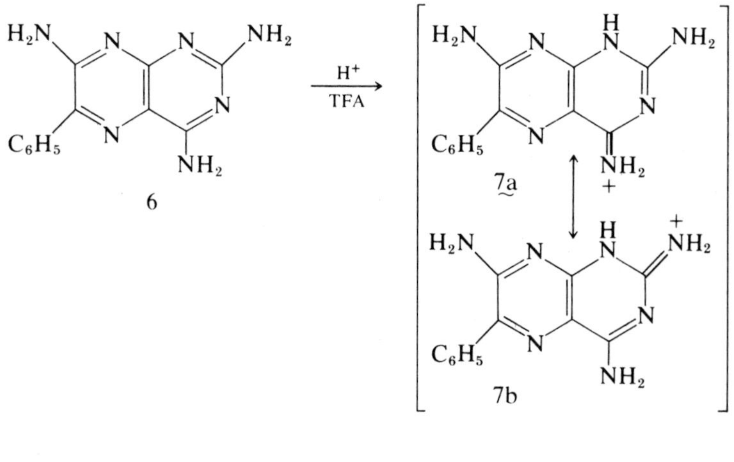

6

7a

7b

Perhaps the result of greatest biological significance is the finding that the positive charge in amiloride is delocalized on the terminal amidinium fragment of the guanidinium moiety. This finding, coupled with the cited conformational results, provides a solid molecular basis upon which to rationally explain the clinically observed qualitative similarities in the antikaliuretic natriuretic profiles displayed by amiloride and triamterene (*Goldberg*, 1973), as well as their demonstrated ability to bind competitively to the same receptors in cells isolated from the bladders of toads, *Bufo marinus* (*Cuthbert* and *Shum*, 1975). Although triamterene displays a pKa of 6.2 and therefore is a weaker base than amiloride, it nevertheless is likely to exist, at least in part, as a cationic species at physiological pH, particularly within the kidney nephron. Protonation of triamterene, 6, is calculated by the CNDO/2 method to most likely occur on the 1-position of the pteridine nucleus (*Gund*, unpublished results). Protonation on N-1, in turn, would give rise to resonance forms 7a and 7b, as shown below (Equation 2), in agreement with previous NMR results (*Weinstock et al.*, 1968) determined for 6 in trifluoroacetic acid. Hence, amiloride and triamterene share two common structural features: a) a structural moiety whose basicity is sufficient to render it a cation at physiological pH, and b) a lipophilic substitutent located at a nuclear site remote to the site of protonation. On the other hand, the ground-state structure of amiloride F1 and the protonated triamterene resonance forms 7a and 7b are not superimposable and, accordingly, it is not surprising that the two drugs neither display equipotent antikaliuretic natriuretic activity nor bind to isolated toad-bladder cells with the same affinity. In both instances, amiloride is clearly the more potent agent.

In conclusion, the simultaneous use of NMR and CNDO/2 methods proved to be a fruitful means for gaining insights into the tautomerism and conformation of amiloride and its free-base form, compounds rendered challenging for study to theoretician and spectroscopist alike by virtue of their structural complexities and physical properties.

REFERENCES

Baer, J.E., and Beyer, K.H., Jr.   1972.   Drugs Affecting Kidney Function and Metabolism. In *Progress in Biochemical Pharmacology*, vol. VII, ed. K.D.G. Edwards. pp. 59–93. Basel: Karger

Benos, D.J., Simon, S.A., Mandel, L.J., and Cala, P.M.   1976.   Effect of amiloride and some of its analogues on cation transport in isolated frog skin and thin lipid membranes. J. Gen. Physiol 68:43–63

Bicking, J.B., Mason, J.W., Woltersdorf, O.W., Jr., Jones, J.H., Kwong, S.F., Robb, C.M., and Cragoe, E.J., Jr.   1965.   Pyrazine diuretics I. N-amidino-3-amino-6-halopyrazinecarboxamides: J Med Chem 8:638–642

Burge, P.S., and Montuschi, E. 1976. Long-term effects of an amiloride/hydrochlorothiazide combination (MODURETIC) on electrolyte balance. Curr Med Res Opin 4:260–262

Cuthbert, A.W., and Shum, W.K. 1975. Effects of vasopressin and aldosterone on amiloride binding in toad bladder epithelial cells. Proc R Soc Lond B 189:543–575

Cuthbert, A.W. 1976. Importance of guanidinium groups for blocking sodium channels in epithelia. Mol Pharmacol 12:945–957

Ganellin, C.R. 1977. Chemical Constitution and Prototropic Equilibria in Structure-Activity Analysis. In *Drug Action at the Molecular Level*, G.C.K. Roberts. pp. 1–39. ed. Baltimore-London-Tokyo: University Park Press

Glitzer, M.S., Steelman, S.L. 1966. N-amidino-3,5-diamino-6-chloropyrazinecarboxamide; An active diuretic in the carboxamide series. Nature 212:191–193

Goldberg, M. 1973. The Renal Physiology of Diuretics. In: Handbook of Physiology, Section 8: Renal Physiology, p. 1003. Washington, D.C.: American Physiology Society

Gund, P. unpublished results.

Hirshfield, J., Springer, J., and Hoogsteen, K. unpublished results.

Matsumoto, K., Rappoport, H. 1968. The preparation and properties of some acylguanidines. J Org Chem 33:552–558

Schapel, G.J., Edwards, K.D.G., and Robinson, J. 1975. Potassium-sparing effect of amiloride in a diuretic factorial study in man. Clin Exp Pharmacol Physiol 2:277–287

Smith, R.L., Cochran, D.W., Gund, P., and Cragoe, E.J., Jr. Proton, Carbon-13 and Nitrogen-15 nuclear magnetic resonance and CNDO/2 studies on the tautomerism and conformation of amiloride, a novel acylguanidine. J. Am Chem Soc, in press

Stearns, J.F., and Rappoport, H. 1977. Reduction of acylguanidines to alkylguanidines with lithium aluminum hydride. J Org Chem 42:3608–3614

Stoner, L.C., Burg, M.R., and Orloff, J. 1974. Ion transport in cortical collecting tubule; effect of amiloride. Am J Physiol 227:453–459

Weinstock, J., Dunoff, R.F., Sutton, B., Trost, B., Kirkpatrick, J., Farnia, F., and Straub, A.S. 1968. Pteridines. VI. Preparation of some 6-aryl-7-aminopteridines. J Med Chem 11:549–556

The Comparative Pharmacology of Amiloride

P. J. Bentley

Departments of Pharmacology and Ophthalmology
Mt. Sinai School of Medicine of
The City University of New York
New York, New York 10029

The development of amiloride is a notable example of the application of applied research to the development of basic principles. This interesting drug has unquestionably provided a significant landmark in our efforts to understand how ions move across membranes. It has displayed a quite remarkable ability to reversibly inhibit at low concentrations the movement of cations across biological membranes in a wide variety of tissues, organs and species which include not only vertebrates but also invertebrates. Such ubiquitous actions strongly suggest that we are dealing with a basic common entity, or mechanism, concerned with ion transport. Because of this ubiquitous propensity to inhibit ion transport at different sites, amiloride also has provided a tool for studying the interaction of sodium permeability and transport with other types of processes that occur in cells. In this way, amiloride has also entered the hallowed realm of developmental embryology (*Powers, Borland,* and *Biggers,* 1977), which is described later in this volume (*Biggers* and *Powers,* Na$^+$ Transport and Swelling of the Mammalian Blastocyst: Effect of Amiloride). It also has been shown to inhibit the regeneration of limbs in salamanders, apparently by interfering with cutaneous electrical currents that regulate such processes (*Borgens, Vanable,* and *Jaffe,* 1977).

In this presentation the common actions of amiloride in diverse biological sites and species of animals will be described briefly. The details will be found in subsequent papers in this volume.

It was shown in dogs and rats that amiloride promoted urinary sodium loss, but unlike most other diuretics then available, this effect was not accompanied by an increase in excretion of potassium (*Baer et al.,* 1967). It was thus one of the early members of the family of

All of the author's personal work cited in this paper was supported by the National Science Foundation.

potassium-sparing diurectics. Clinical trials soon confirmed that it has a similar action in man (*Bull* and *Laragh*, 1968). Its effect was shown to most probably occur in the nether regions of the renal tubule where it could inhibit the process of reabsorption of sodium. The renal tubule does not readily lend itself to studies of the precise mechanism of action of such drugs; thus, it was rather exciting to find that amiloride also acted on various other epithelial membrane preparations under *in vitro* conditions. In 1967 in Germany *Eigler*, *Kelter*, and *Renner* showed that amiloride inhibited the short-circuit current (SCC, a reflection of active Na transport) across frog skin *in vitro*. The next year similar effects were reported on the urinary bladder of the toad *Bufo marinus* (*Bentley*, 1968; *Ehrlich* and *Crabbé*, 1968). Both the skin and urinary bladder of amphibians are widely considered to provide models for many of the transport processes that occur in the mammalian kidney. It also was shown at this time that amiloride could inhibit the SCC across the colon of *Bufo marinus*. It thus became apparent that the action of amiloride was not confined to kidneys or even to mammals.

The early studies suggested that amiloride was acting on such epithelia to block the access of Na to the Na "pump" so that its action appeared to be a permeability effect. It could inhibit metabolism, but this action is probably indirect and related to the presence of Na (see, for instance, *Parisi* and *Bentley*, 1970).

Apart from common anuran amphibians like frogs and toads, amiloride also has been shown to inhibit Na transport across the skin and urinary bladders of more exotic urodele amphibians, including the mud eel *Siren lacertina* (*Bentley*, 1973, 1975) and the congo eel *Amphiuma means* (*Bentley*, 1973, 1975; *Mullen et al.*, 1976; *Degnan* and *Zadunaisky*. 1977). However, it does not work on the skin of all amphibians; for instance, it is ineffective on the skin of the mudpuppy *Necturus maculous* (*Bentley* and *Yorio*, 1977) but does act on the bladder of that species (*Bentley*, 1971). Mudpuppies are rather exceptional among amphibians, however, as they do not appear to normally actively transport Na across their skin. Yet if one exposes the outer surface of their skin to amphotericin B, an active Na transport develops which can be inhibited by ouabain but is unaffected by amiloride. This failure on the part of amiloride to block the effects of this antibiotic also has been seen in toad urinary bladder (*Bentley*, 1968). These observations are of interest as they show that amiloride cannot block an "old hole" in a membrane. Mudpuppies seem normally to lack specific "Na channels" on which the drug can act. These animals are neotenous (they are really just big tadpoles) and do not seem to have reached the stage of development when such specific cutaneous sites appear. The embryological development of amiloride-sensitive Na channels is described later in this symposium.

Before leaving the amphibia, it should be pointed out that the effects of amiloride are not necessarily specific for Na or apparently even cations. Lithium can cross frog skin and toad urinary bladder (*Herrera*, 1972; *Leblanc* and *Lemonnier*, 1971; *Candia* and *Chiarandini*, 1973), and its movement, like that of Na, is also blocked by amiloride, suggesting that the two ions utilize common pathways.

It was not surprising to observe that reptilian epithelia which transport Na also can respond to amiloride. This effect has been shown in the urinary bladder of the turtle *Pseudemys scripta* (*Wilczewski* and *Brodsky*, 1975). It also inhibits the SCC across the colon of some rather exotic lizards belonging to the genus *Amphibolurus* that live in the deserts of Australia (*Bentley* and *Bradshaw*, 1972). Amiloride recently has been shown to inhibit the Na-dependent PD across the distal renal tubule of the snake *Thamnophis in vitro* (*Beyenbach* and *Dantzler*, 1978). I have been unable to find any reference to its actions in birds, but suspect that the chicken cloaca may be susceptible to its action. Kirschner has shown that amiloride's action can extend even to fish and invertebrates (*Kirschner, Greenwald,* and *Kerstetter*, 1973).

To return to mammals, amiloride also has been shown to have many extrarenal effects in these vertebrates. It thus can inhibit Na transport across the rabbit colon (*Frizzell, Koch,* and *Schultz*, 1976; *Yorio* and *Bentley*, 1977), esophagus (*Powell, Morris,* and *Boyd*, 1975) and urinary bladder (*Lewis* and *Diamond*, 1976). It also blocks the reabsorption of Na from the submaxillary gland of the rat (*Schneyer*, 1970). Generally speaking, the effects of amiloride seem to be confined to epithelial membranes, but there is one interesting observation showing that it blocks passive Na entry into human red cells (*Aceves* and *Cereijido*, 1973). As far as I am aware, this observation is unique. Benos and his collaborators (*Benos et al.*, 1976) have shown that amiloride can increase the surface potential of artificial lipid bilayer membranes prepared from sheep red cell lipids. However, this effect was not specifically related to the pharmacological activity of amiloride and its analogues but appeared to be due to the electrical charge carried by the molecule. Amiloride does not act on all types of epithelia. Thus, it does not appear to inhibit Na transport in the proximal renal tubule (*Duarte, Chomety* and *Giebisch*, 1971) and the choroid plexus (*Wright*, 1972); nor, as far as I am aware, are there any reports of its working on the small intestine or gallbladder. All of these membranes fit into the classification of being low-resistance "leaky" epithelia (*Frömter* and *Diamond*, 1972).

The ubiquitous distribution of the ability of amiloride (see Table 1) to block Na transport across "tight" epithelia raises the question of whether there is a characteristic primeval structural entity which acts as a Na channel in all such animal epithelia. Does it have a divine origin which is a prerequisite for the life of many types of multicellular

Table 1.   Phyletic Distribution of Responses to Amiloride in Tetrapods

Target Tissue	Source
Mammals	
Renal tubule	*Baer et al.*, 1967
Esophagus	*Powell, Morris,* and *Boyd,* 1975
Colon	*Frizzell, Koch,* and *Schultz,* 1976; *Yorio* and *Bentley,* 1977
Urinary bladder	*Lewis* and *Diamond,* 1976
Submaxillary gland	*Schneyer,* 1970
Erythrocytes	*Aceves* and *Cereijido,* 1973
Reptiles	
Turtle urinary bladder	*Wilczewski and Brodsky,* 1975
Lizard Colon	*Bentley* and *Bradshaw,* 1972
Snake Kidney	*Beyenbach* and *Dantzler,* 1978
Birds	
?	
Amphibia	
a. Anura	
Skin	*Eigler, Kelter,* and *Renner,* 1967
Urinary bladder	*Bentley,* 1968; *Ehrlich* and *Crabbé,* 1968
Colon	*Bentley,* 1968; *Ehrlich* and *Crabbé,* 1968
b. Urodela	
Skin	*Bentley,* 1973, 1975
Urinary bladder	*Bentley,* 1971, 1973, 1975; *Mullen et al.,* 1976; *Degnan* and *Zadunaisky,* 1977

organisms? The widespread effectiveness of amiloride suggests that such Na channels could at least have an inherent basic similarity throughout the animal kingdom. However, it should be recalled that other types of Na channels exist, e.g., as in nerve and muscle, and these characteristically can be blocked by tetrodotoxin. There does not, however, appear to be any significant crossover in the sensitivity of each type of channel to the two types of drugs, though both possess a guanidinium moiety which appears to be essential for their actions. One is immediately tempted to question the nature of the differences in these two types of sodium channels. Most likely, such problems will be ultimately resolved only if or when they can be isolated and chemically characterized. Judging from the recent success in isolating "receptors," which is possibly all that the Na channel really is, this may be feasible and occur sooner than many of us suspect. Amiloride promises to be useful for the labeling of such channels.

REFERENCES

Aceves, J. and Cereijido, M.   1973.   The effect of amiloride on sodium and potassium fluxes in red cells. J Physiol Lond 229:709–718

Baer, J.E., Jones, C.B., Spitzer, S.A. and Russo, H.F. 1967. The potassium-sparing and natriuretic activity of N-amidino-3,5-diamino-6-chloro-pyrazinecarboxyamide hydrochloride dihydrate (Amiloride hydrochloride). J Pharm Exp Therap 157:472–485

Benos, D.J., Simon, S.A., Mandel, L.J. and Cala, P.M. 1976. Effect of amiloride and some of its analogues on cation transport in isolated frog skin and thin lipid membranes. J Gen Physiol 68:43–63.

Bentley, P.J. 1968. Amiloride: A potent inhibitor of sodium transport across the toad bladder. J Physiol Lond 195:317–330

Bentley, P.J. 1971. Sodium and water movement across the urinary bladder of a urodele amphibian (the mudpuppy *Necturus maculosus*). Studies with vasotocin and aldosterone. Gen Comp Endocrin 16:356–362

Bentley, P.J. 1973. Osmoregulation in the aquatic urodeles *Amphiuma means* (the congo eel) and *Siren lacertina* (the mud eel). Effects of vasotocin. Gen Comp Endocrin 20:386–391

Bentley, P.J. 1975. The electrical P.D. across the integument of some neotenous urodele amphibians. Comp Biochem Physiol 50A:639–643

Bentley, P.J. and Bradshaw, S.D. 1972. Electrical potential difference across the cloaca and colon of the Australian lizards *Amphibolurus ornatus* and *A. inermis*. Comp Biochem Physiol 42A:465–471

Bentley, P.J. and Yorio, T. 1977. The permeability of the skin of a neotenous urodele amphibian, the mudpuppy *Necturus maculosus*. J Physiol Lond 265:537–547

Beyenbach, K.W. and Dantzler, W.H. 1978. Generation of transepithelial potentials by isolated perfused reptilian distal tubules. Am J Physiol 234:F238–F246

Borgens, R.B., Vanable, J.W. and Jaffe, L.F. 1977. Skin current and regeneration. Amer Zoologist 17:867

Bull, M.B. and Laragh, J.H. 1968. Amiloride. A potassium-sparing natriuretic agent. Circulation 37:45–53

Candia, O.A. and Chiarandini, D.J. 1973. Transport of lithium and rectification by frog skin. Biochem Biophys Acta 307:578–589

Degnan, K.J. and Zadunaisky, J.A. 1977. The electrical properties and active ion transport across the urinary bladder of the urodele, *Amphiuma means*. J Physiol Lond 265:207–230

Duarte, C., Chomety, F. and Giebisch, G. 1971. Effect of amiloride, ouabain, and furosemide on distal tubular function in the rat. Am J Physiol 221:632–639

Ehrlich, E.N. and Crabbé, J. 1968. The mechanism of action of amipramizide. Pflügers Arch 302:79–96

Eigler, J., Kelter, J. and Renner, E. 1967. Wirkungscharakteristika eines neuen Acylguanidins- Amiloride-HCl (Mk-870)-an der isolierten Haut von Amphibien. Klin Wochenschr 45:737–738

Frizzell, R.A., Koch, M.J. and Schultz, S.G. 1976. Ion transport by rabbit colon. I. Active and passive components. J Membrane Biol 27:297–316

Frömter, E. and Diamond, J. 1972. Route of passive ion permeation in epithelia. Nature, New Biology 235:9–13

Herrera, F.C. 1972 Inhibition of lithium transport across toad bladder by amiloride. Am J Physiol 222:499–502

Kirschner, L.B., Greenwald, L. and Kerstetter, T.H. 1973. Effect of amiloride on sodium transport across body surfaces of freshwater animals. Am J Physiol 224:832–837

Leblanc, G. and Lemonnier, R. 1971. Lithium uptake by isolated epithelium from frog skin and its inhibition by amiloride. Proc Int Union of Physiol Sci LX:339

Lewis, S.A. and Diamond, J.M. 1976. Na$^+$ transport by rabbit urinary bladder, a tight epithelium. J Membrane Biol 28:1–40

Mullen, J.L., Kashgarian, M., Biemesderfer, D., Giebisch, G.H. and Biber, T.U.L. 1976. Ion transport and structure of urinary bladder epithelium of *Amphiuma*. Am J Physiol 231:501–508

Parisi, M. and Bentley, P.J. 1970 Effects of amiloride on respiration of the urinary bladder, intestine and sartorius muscle of toads. Biochim Biophys Acta 219:234–237

Powell, D.W., Morris, S.M. and Boyd, D.D. 1975. Water and electrolyte transport by rabbit esophagus. Am J Physiol 229:438–443

Powers, R.D., Borland, R.M. and Biggers, J.D. 1977. Amiloride-sensitive rheogenic Na$^+$ transport in rabbit blastocyst. Nature Lond 270:603–604

Schneyer, L.H. 1970. Amiloride inhibition of ion transport in perfused excretory duct of rat submaxillary gland. Am J Physiol 219:1050–1055

Wilczewski, T. and Brodsky, W.A. 1975. Effects of ouabain and amiloride on Na pathways in turtle bladders. Am J Physiol 228:781–790

Wright, E.M. 1972. Mechanisms of ion transport across the choroid plexus. J Physiol Lond 226:545–571

Yorio, T. and Bentley, P.J. 1977. Permeability of the rabbit colon *in vitro*. Am J Physiol 232:F5–F9

Extrarenal Action of Amiloride in Aquatic Animals

Leonard B. Kirschner

Department of Zoology
Washington State University
Pullman, Washington 99163

Shortly after its introduction as a natriuretic, diuretic agent, amiloride was shown to block active Na^+ transport across isolated frog skin (*Eigler, Kelter*, and *Renner*, 1967) and toad bladder (*Bentley*, 1968). During the past decade similar observations have been made on many extrarenal organs in both vertebrate and invertebrate animals. This paper reviews some aspects of amiloride's action on sodium transport across the body surface of intact, freshwater (FW) animals and considers one implication of this action for the evolution of the transport systems.

The first detailed study on intact animals was carried on in trout (*Kirschner*, 1973). This was later extended to frogs and crayfish (*Kirschner, Greenwald*, and *Kerstetter*, 1973). Figure 1 shows inhibition of undirectional Na^+ influx across trout gill when amiloride was added to the external medium. The action was rapidly and completely reversible. It was also shown to be specific for the Na transport system. Chloride uptake, also by active transport in the intact animal, was unaffected, as shown in Figure 2. Indeed, amiloride has been one of the tools used to show that Na^+ and Cl^- transport systems are independent of each other. Inhibition of sodium transport also has been shown in two FW annelids (*Kirschner, Greenwald*, and *Kerstetter*, 1973; *Dietz* and *Alvarado*, 1970) and in a mussel (*Dietz*, in press), as well as in a number of other FW vertebrates.

It was mentioned above that both Na^+ and Cl^- are actively transported inward in intact animals, and that the two transport systems

The research described was supported by grants GM-02454 and GM-01276 from the National Institute of General Medical Sciences. The author is indebted to Dr. Thomas Dietz for providing unpublished data on the dose-response relationship for the earthworm *Lumbricus terrestris* and the mussel *Carunculina texasensis*.

41

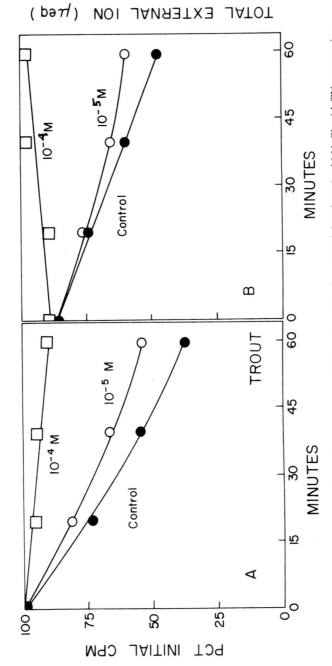

Fig. 1.   Effect of amiloride on sodium influx across trout gill. The external medium containing about 1 mM NaCl, with ^{22}Na, was recirculated across the gills of anesthetized fish as described by *Kerstetter, Kirschner,* and *Rafuse* (1970). A) Disappearance of ^{22}Na provides a measure of influx from medium into the animal. B) Decrease in total Na provides a measure of net influx. From *Kirschner*, Am J Physiol 224:832–837, 1973.

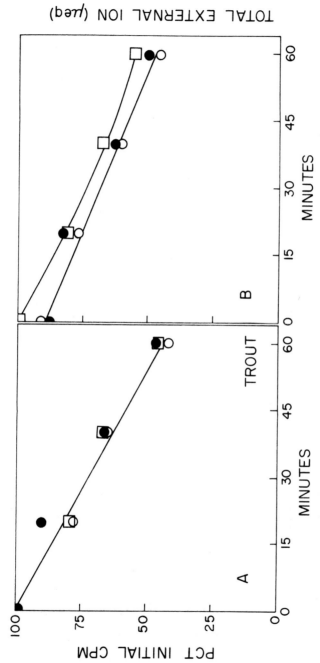

Fig. 2.   Lack of amiloride effect on chloride influx across trout gill. Protocol as for Figure 1, except that the isotope used was ^{36}Cl. From *Kirschner*, Am J Physiol 224:832–837, 1973.

are completely independent of each other in most cases. This can be possible only if, for example, the uptake of Na^+ is accompanied by an equivalent excretion of another cation. Such exchanges have been amply demonstrated in many animals, beginning with the classical studies of *Krogh* (1939). There has been some disagreement recently on whether the exchange partner is NH_4^+, H^+, or both (e.g., *Kerstetter, Kirschner,* and *Rafuse,* 1970; *Maetz, Payan,* and *deRenzis,* 1976); but there is general agreement that exchange occurs. Figures 3 and 4 show this for the trout and crayfish. In control animals there is net Na uptake from the dilute medium, because undirectional influx exceeds efflux. The excretion of $NH_4^+ + H^+$ (shown positive in the figures, although it is an efflux) is about the same as net sodium uptake in the crayfish and exceeds it in the trout. Addition of amiloride sharply reduces the influx of Na^+ with little effect on efflux. This is accompanied by a sharp reduction in acid excretion. The nature of the coupling is not known, but data such as these have led to a transport model, such as the one shown in Figure 5, where the apical membrane contains an amiloride-sensitive system exchanging Na^+ for H^+ (and/or NH_4^+) and a second system, insensitive to amiloride, exchanging Cl^- for HCO_3^-. If correct, this means that ionic regulation by these epithelia is intimately connected with acid-base regu-

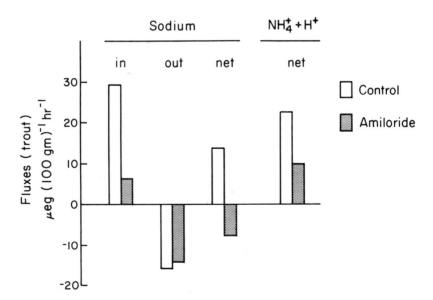

Fig. 3. Sodium fluxes and excretion of H^+ and NH_4^+ across trout gill. The experimental procedure was similar to that used in the previous experiments, except that the medium contained Na_2HPO_4/NaH_2PO_4 (pH ~ 7.2). Fluxes were estimated as described in *Kirschner,* 1973.

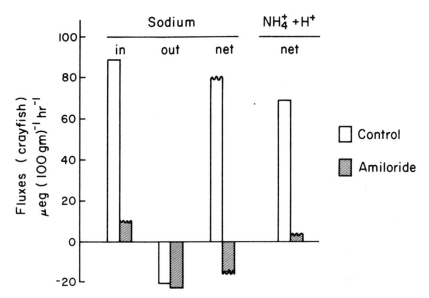

Fig. 4.   Sodium fluxes and excretion of H^+ and NH_4^+ across crayfish gill.

lation. One implication of this interrelationship will be explored further below.

The action of amiloride in intact animals resembles that on isolated epithelia in a number of important ways, notably in site of action, specificity and reversibility. However, there are both quantitative and qualitative differences. First, *Bentley's* 1968 study suggested that the action of amiloride on toad bladder involved more than simple competition with Na for sites on the apical membrane. A more detailed examination, using isolated frog skin, led to a similar conclusion (*Benos et al.*, 1976). Yet

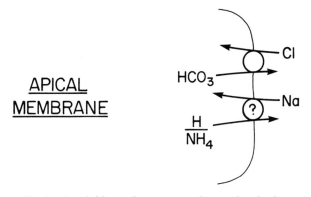

Fig. 5.   Coupled ion exchange systems in aquatic animals.

Figure 6 indicates that competition may well be involved in intact trout. These experiments are technically difficult to carry out *in vivo*, and the conclusion must be considered tentative; but the data provide no indication that a more complex mechanism plays a role under these conditions.

A second difference between *in vivo* and *in vitro* experiments involves effective amiloride concentrations. Figure 7 shows the concentration dependence in representatives from four phyla, and it is clear that all have approximately the same sensitivity (50% inhibition at about 5×10^{-5} M). This range of concentrations is much higher than in isolated epithelia (*Benos et al.*, 1976). The difference is especially striking in that Na^+ concentrations are much lower in these experiments (about 1 mM) than in experiments on isolated preparations (about 100 mM). If there is competition between amiloride and Na^+ for negatively charged groups on the apical surface, it might have been predicted that the inhibitor would be more rather than less effective at low Na concentrations *in vivo*, as is the case *in vitro* (*Cuthbert* and *Shum*, 1974). Finally, amiloride inhibition in isolated frog skin is strongly dependent on the

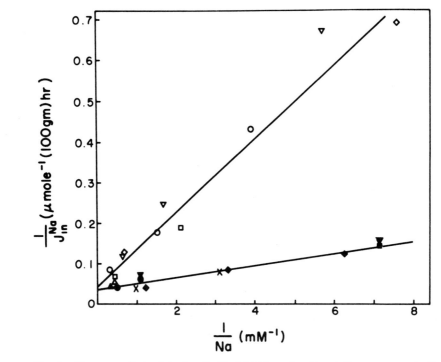

Fig. 6.   Lineweaver-Burk plot of amiloride inhibition of sodium influx across trout gill. The experiment is described in *Kirschner, Greenwald*, and *Kerstetter*, J Membrane Biol 26:371–383, 1976.

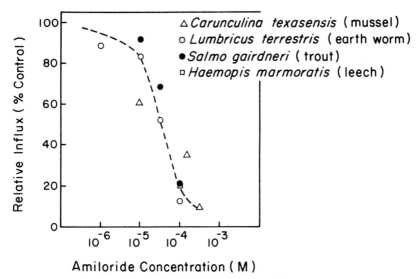

Fig. 7.   Concentration dependence of amiloride inhibition. The data for different animals were obtained in several laboratories. Conditions varied slightly, but the methods were variants of those in Figure 1.

presence of calcium (*Cuthbert* and *Wong*, 1972), whereas the action on intact animals, including the frog, is independent of ambient calcium (*Kirschner, Greenwald*, and *Kerstetter*, 1973).

We have also examined a number of other amino compounds and found that lysine methyl ester (MeL) also is inhibitory when added to the external medium. Figure 8 shows an experiment in which 5 mM MeL reduced Na^+ uptake across trout gill. Its action was similar to that of amiloride in specificity and reversibility, but a much higher concentration was required (1–10 mM). Thus, 10 mM MeL depressed Na influx to about 45% of the control (N = 7), with no effect on Na or Cl effluxes. Lysine was not inhibitory; in fact, it stimulated Na transport. Methyl esters of monoamino acids also were ineffective.

The action of amiloride in FW animals from several phyla raises another question worth exploring, one with evolutionary overtones. Any FW animal must regulate internal Na above ambient and therefore must be able to absorb it against an electrochemical potential gradient. In all complex metazoans the transport system is incorporated into an epithelium bathed on the apical side by the medium and on the basolateral side by the extracellular fluids (ECF). The "Na transport system" thus comprises at least two steps: one transferring Na from a dilute medium into the cell, the second moving it from cell to ECF. A model of the first step, synthesized from data on many animals, is shown in Figure 5. Perhaps

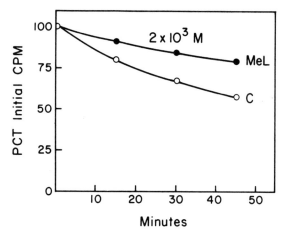

Fig. 8. Methyl-lysine inhibition of sodium influx across trout gill. An experiment as shown in Figure 1.

the most striking feature is amiloride sensitivity, for the ability of this compound to block transport in all FW animals examined thus far seems to imply that the molecular structure of the transfer system is similar in all of them. Such a widespread distribution argues for early development of the molecular machinery and only minor modification during evolution. However, this means that the amiloride-sensitive step cannot have evolved as an adaptation to FW, because the invasion of FW by major taxonomic groups certainly took place independently, each from marine ancestors in the same group. Instead, one must look to the earliest appearance of such a system in a marine environment. If so, it cannot have been in conjunction with active Na^+ uptake; nearly all marine invertebrates are at virtual ionic equilibrium with the NaCl in seawater. The few marine animals that are not at equilibrium (e.g., modern fish) must extrude, not absorb, Na^+; hence they provide no clue.

One characteristic shared by all aquatic animals is the need to excrete H^+ and NH_3. This requirement is probably as old as heterotrophic metabolism. It recently has been proposed (*Evans*, 1975) that catalyzed Na^+ uptake coupled to excretion of H^+ and/or NH_4^+ may have developed as a means for accelerating the removal of these metabolic end products across the body surface. This would explain why an apical Na^+ transfer system might appear in marine animals that had no need to absorb this ion. An early appearance followed by conservation of molecular details during evolution would result in widespread occurrence at a later time. Moreover, the existence of such a system in marine animals would "preadapt" them for invading FW. That is, even though the mechanism developed to accelerate metabolite excretion, the ability to move Na$^+$ in through the apical membrane would permit marine animals to invade more dilute media in which active uptake became necessary in order to maintain ECF ion concentrations above ambient. It is difficult to test such an historical proposition. However, if it is correct, one might expect to find amiloride-sensitive, coupled Na$^+$/H$^+$ + NH$_4$$^+$ exchange systems widespread among modern marine invertebrates, even through they are isoionic with the NaCl in seawater.

REFERENCES

Benos, D.J., Simon, S.A., Mandel, L.J., and Cala, P.M. 1976. Effect of amiloride and some of its analogues on cation transport in isolated frog skin and thin lipid membranes. J Gen Physiol 68:43–63

Bentley, P.J. 1968 Amiloride: A potent inhibitor of sodium transport across the toad bladder. J Physiol (London) 195:317–330

Cuthbert, A.W. and Wong, P.Y.D. 1972. The role of calcium ions in the interaction of amiloride with membrane receptors. Mol Pharmacol 8:222–229

Cuthbert, A.W. Shum, W.K. 1974. Amiloride and the sodium channel. Arch Pharmacol 281:261–269

Dietz, T.H. 1978. Sodium transport in the freshwater mussel, *Carunculina texasensis*. Amer J Physiol 235:R35–R40

Dietz, T.H. and Alvarado, R.H. 1970. Osmotic and ionic regualtion in *Lumbricus terrestris*. Biol Bull 138:247–261

Eigler, J., Kelter, J. and Renner, E. 1967. Wirkungscharakteristik eines neuen Acylguanadins-amiloride-HCL an der isolierten Haut von Amphibien. Klin Wochenschr 43:737–738

Evans, D.H. 1975. Ionic exchange mechanisms in fish gills. Comp Biochem Physiol 51A:491–495

Greenwald, L.E. and Kirschner, L.B. 1976. The effect of poly-L-lysine, amiloride and methyl-L-lysine on gill ion transport and permeability in the rainbow trout. J Membrane Biol 26:371–383

Kerstetter, T.H., Kirschner, L.B. and Rafuse, D.D. 1970. On the mechanisms of sodium transport by the irrigated gills of rainbow trout. J Gen Physiol 56:342–359

Kirschner, L.B. 1973. Electrolyte transport across body surfaces of freshwater fish and amphibia. In Transport Mechanisms in Epithelia, Alfred Benzon Symposium, V. eds. H.H. Ussing, and N.A. Thorn. pp.447–460, Copenhagen:Munksgaard.

Kirschner, L.B., Greenwald, L. and Kerstetter, T.H. 1973. Effect of amiloride on sodium transport across body surfaces of freshwater animals. Amer J Physiol 224:832–837

Krogh, A. 1939. Osmotic Regulation in Aquatic Animals. London: Cambridge University Press.

Maetz, J., Payan, P., and deRenzis, G. 1976. Controversial aspects of ionic uptake in freshwater animals. In Perspectives in Experimental Zoology, ed P.S. Davies, London: Pergammon Press.

©1979 Urban & Schwarzenberg, Inc. Baltimore-Munich
Amiloride and Epithelial Sodium Transport
Edited by A.W. Cuthbert, G.M. Fanelli, Jr. and A. Scriabine

Studies with Amiloride on Isolated Distal Nephron Segments

Larry C. Stoner

Department of Physiology
Upstate Medical Center
State University of New York
Syracuse, New York 13210

INTRODUCTION

The pyrazine diuretic, amiloride, administered to dog, rat, or man (*Baer et al.*, 1967; *Bull* and *Laragh*, 1968; *Guignard* and *Peters*, 1970), results in modest increases in the urinary excretion of sodium, while causing a striking reduction in the excretion of potassium. The inhibition of potassium excretion, together with the relatively small magnitude of the natriuresis, has been taken to indicate that the site of action of this drug is somewhere in the distal nephron. Clearance, stop-flow and micropuncture studies all support this conclusion (*Baer et al.*, 1967; *Bull* and *Laragh*, 1968).

Most of the distal nephron is located deep in the renal mass and is inaccessible to direct assessment by micropuncture. Hypotheses regarding the mechanism of action of amiloride are largely derived from its effects on frog skin (*Dörge* and *Nagel*, 1970), and toad bladder (*Bentley*, 1968; *Ehrlich* and *Crabbé*, 1968). In these epithelia amiloride causes a rapid, reversible inhibition of active sodium transport and the associated spontaneous transepithelial potential difference. Investigators have observed an increase in the specific resistance of these epithelia when amiloride was administered (*Dörge* and *Nagel*, 1970; *Ehrlich* and *Crabbé*, 1968). These observations have led to a simple model for the drug's effect. Reduction of the permeability of the mucosal membrane of the epithelial cell to sodium by amiloride prevents the entry of sodium into the mucosal or apical border of the cell. A lowered intracellular sodium presumably deprives the active transport mechanism, located at the serosal or basal membrane, of sodium for transport.

The development of the techniques of the *in vitro* perfusion of fragments of the rabbit nephron in 1966 by Burg and associates at the National Institutes of Health (*Burg et al.*, 1966) has permitted a direct assessment of the transport properties of nephron segments located deep in the renal mass. In its simplest form, the technique involves suspension of a nephron fragment (usually dissected from the rabbit) between pairs of concentric glass pipets. At the perfusion end of the tubule fluid is forced into the lumen either by gravity or a perfusion pump. This fluid can then be collected with a sampling pipet at the collecting end of the tubule fragment. The ability to analyze the chemical or radioisotopic content of the collected fluid permits us to assess the transport processes of the tubule segment. The spontaneous transepithelial voltage at the perfusion end of the epithelium can be recorded by using the inner perfusion pipet as an electrode. Finally, the ability to inject a small current allows estimation of the electrical conductance of this epithelium. These bioelectric parameters have long been held as important indices of ion transport.

Four segments of the rabbit nephron have been studied with respect to their sensitivity to the potassium-sparing diuretic, amiloride. They are: a) the cortical thick ascending limb of Henle's loop; b) the distal convoluted tubule, which is defined as that portion of the nephron extending from the macula densa to the first branch of a collecting tubule; c) the granular cortical collecting tubule; and d) the light portion of the cortical collecting tubule. As recently described by *Morel*, *Chabardes*, and *Imbert* (1976), the granular cortical collecting tubule is readily distinguished from the light portion of the cortical collecting tubule on the basis of its larger tubular diameter and the "granular" appearance of the cells.

The studies of *Burg* and *Green* (1973) demonstrated that the thick ascending limb of Henle reabsorbs sodium chloride by a unique mechanism. They observed that the transepithelial voltage was oriented positive in the lumen. This was taken as evidence that chloride absorption was against an electrochemical gradient and must be an active process. Experiments designed to test the mechanism of net sodium absorption in this segment led to the conclusion that it moves passively down its electrical gradient (*Burg* and *Green*, 1973).

Data in Table 1 show that amiloride at 10^{-4} M, placed in both the bath and perfusate solutions, results in little or no effect on either the transepithelial potential difference or the net lumen-to-bath flux of chloride across the thick ascending limb. Also shown in Table 1 is the effect of 10^{-5} M furosemide. This diuretic inhibits about 80% of both the spontaneous voltage and the rate of net chloride absorption.

Table 1.   Effect of Diuretics on the Thick Ascending
Limb of Henle

Condition	Spontaneous Voltage (mV)	Net Chloride Absorption Rate (pM mm^{-1} min^{-1})
Control	+5.8 mV	56
Amiloride (10^{-4} M)	+5.4 mV	54
Furosemide (10^{-5} M)	+1.0 mV	13

Amiloride was applied to both lumen and bath. Furosemide
placed in perfusate only. Data modified from *Burg* and *Green*
(1973) and *Stoner, Burg,* and *Orloff* (1974).

The second segment studied was the light portion of the cortical
collecting tubule. This nephron fragment exhibits ion transport properties
that are strikingly different from those of the thick ascending limb. In
this tubule segment sodium and not chloride appears to be the actively
transported ion species. Table 2 presents a Ussing analysis of the
transport of both sodium and potassium across the light cortical collecting tubule. The unidirectional fluxes (lumen-to-bath and bath-to-lumen)
of ^{24}Na$^+$ and ^{42}K$^+$ were measured in a series of collecting tubules. The
potential difference necessary to produce the flux ratio (the lumen-to-
bath flux divided by the bath-to-lumen flux) by passive diffusion was calculated using the Ussing equation (*Ussing*, 1952). The average spontaneous voltage of these tubules was -35 mV, lumen-negative. Sodium
absorption cannot be a passive process since it would require a spontaneous lumen-positive voltage of nearly $+50$ mV. To postulate that
potassium secretion is passive down its electrical gradient, a lumen-negative -59 mV would be required. Given an observed potential difference
of -35 mV, we have concluded that potassium secretion is at least in
part an active process. *Grantham, Burg,* and *Orloff* (1970) have drawn
similar conclusions for the mechanism of sodium and potassium

Table 2.   Unidirectional Ion Fluxes Across Rabbit Cortical Collecting Tubules

Ion	(n)	Unidirectional Flux (pM mm^{-1} min^{-1}) Lumen-to-bath	Bath-to-lumen	Flux Ratio	E_i(mV)
Sodium	(15)	61.2	9.0	6.8	+48
Potassium	(8)	0.84	9.66	0.09	-59

Data modified from *Stoner, Burg,* and *Orloff* (1974).

transport across the collecting tubule using the Nernst relationship. Thus, the properties of voltage and active sodium transport are similar to those reported for other epithelial systems known to be amiloride-sensitive (*Bentley*, 1968; *Dörge* and *Nagel*, 1970; *Ehrlich* and *Crabbé*, 1968).

The net fluxes of sodium, potassium and chloride and the trans-epithelial voltage are presented in Table 3. These transport data were obtained by measuring the unidirectional radioisotopic fluxes across the tubule, the difference being the net flux. Sodium is absorbed from the tubule lumen at a rate of 52 pM mm^{-1} min^{-1}. Potassium is secreted into the lumen; secretion is denoted here as a negative net lumen-to-bath flux. While not presented in this table, the net flux of Cl has also been measured. The rate of chloride movement was 37.2 pM mm^{-1} min^{-1}, a value roughly equal to the difference between Na absorption and K secretion. The potential difference across this tubule segment is 35 mV, negative in the lumen.

Amiloride at 10^{-5} in the perfusate caused an abolition of the normally lumen-negative voltage, as shown in Table 3. The voltage actually becomes lumen-positive after administration of amiloride. This effect is readily reversible. It is a very rapid effect, occurring as quickly as one can change the solution, a process which requires only a few seconds. This concentration of amiloride also affects the active transport of sodium and potassium of the cortical collecting tubule, as shown in Table 3. In this group of tubules active sodium transport was reduced from 52.2 to 5.4 pM mm^{-1}, min^{-1}, an inhibition of about 90%. Active potassium secretion was reduced to about 5% of its control level. Amiloride also caused a marked increase in the specific resistance of the light cortical collecting tubule (Table 3). *O'Neil* and *Helman* (1977) recently have reported similar observations.

Table 3. Effect of Amiloride on Ion Transport (Lumen-to-Bath) Across the Rabbit Cortical Collecting Tubule

	Control Value	Amiloride (10^{-5} M in lumen)
Voltage (mV)	−35	+5
Specific Resistance (Ω cm^2)	266	358
Ion Flux (pM mm^{-1} min^{-1})		
J_{Na}	52.2	5.4
$J_K{}^+$	−13.2	−0.6

Data modified from *Stoner*, *Burg*, and *Orloff* (1974).

Table 4. Effect of Amiloride or Furosemide on the
Voltage Across the Rabbit Distal Convoluted Tubule

DCT	Transepithelial Potential Difference (mV)			
	Control	Furosemide	Control	Amiloride
1	+7.2	+2.1	+4.2	+3.7
2	+4.6	+0.3	+3.8	+3.7
3	−20.1	−17.6	−17.1	−4.3
4	−5.5	−5.2	−4.9	0.0
5	−3.9	−5.3	—	+0.3

Inhibition of the spontaneous voltage and active sodium transport concomitant with an increase in specific resistance are similar to the reported effects of amiloride on the frog skin and toad bladder. These effects are consistent with the simple model of drug action already stated. A reduced permeability of the luminal membrane to sodium (reflected by an increase in transepithelial resistance) ultimately reduces active sodium transport.

We also have studied the effects of amiloride on the rabbit distal convoluted tubule. Dr. Shareghi, who until recently was a member of my laboratory, was responsible for most of the experiments.

The distal convoluted tubule is conventionally defined as that portion of the nephron which extends from the macula densa to the first branching of the collecting tree. In recent years several laboratories have presented either histological or physiological evidence suggesting that this nephron segment is functionally heterogeneous along its length. Some of the transport characteristics of the rabbit distal convoluted tubule and the effects of placing either 5×10^{-5} M amiloride or furosemide (*Burg et al.*, 1973) in the perfusate are presented in Table 4. Observed values for the transepithelial voltage are presented for each of the five tubules studied. In tubules 1 and 2 the tip of the inner perfusion pipet, which is used to record the potential difference, was within 100 microns of the macula densa, clearly the early distal convoluted tubule. The spontaneous voltages recorded here were lumen-positive. Tubules 3 and 4 were perfused retrograde so that the potential recorded is that of the late distal convoluted tubule. Here the voltage was found to be lumen-negative. Tubule 5 was perfused in the same direction as the first two, except that the initial third of the tubule was damaged in dissection and was cut away before perfusion. The small negative voltage observed represents a value for the mid-distal convoluted tubule. In the two tubules studied, furosemide dramatically reduced the lumen-positive voltage observed in the early distal convoluted tubule. In those tubules where a negative voltage was recorded from the late distal convoluted tubule, this drug appeared to have little or no effect. In contrast, amiloride had no significant effect on the positive voltage of the early distal convoluted tubule but greatly reduced the negative voltage seen in the later portions of this nephron segment.

The effects of these diuretic drugs on sodium absorption and potassium secretion are presented in Table 5. The mean control values for sodium absorption and potassium secretion by these tubules were 82.3 and 9.3 pM mm^{-1} min^{-1}, respectively. Furosemide reduced the sodium absorption by nearly 50%, while potassium secretion appeared to increase slightly. The standard errors here are such that this apparent increase is not significant. After the removal of furosemide, amiloride was added to the perfusate. In each case amiloride reduced the rate of sodium absorption by about 60% and the potassium secretion to 15% of its control value. We conclude from these data that the rabbit distal convoluted tubule has at least two functionally distinct units: the early distal convoluted tubule which exhibits a lumen-positive voltage, and the late distal tubule which exhibits a lumen-negative voltage. While other experiments will be necessary to differentiate the specific site of amiloride action within the distal convoluted tubule, we postulate that the early distal tubule has properties similar to those of the thick ascending of Henle's loop: sodium chloride absorption secondary to furosemide-sensitive active chloride transport. The more distal portions of this segment may reabsorb sodium actively and secrete potassium, properties similar to those of the cortical collecting tubule. Presumably, it is this portion of the tubule that is sensitive to the diuretic amiloride.

Barratt et al. (1975) recently reported a potential profile along the rat distal convoluted tubule similar to that presented here. They observed positive values for the early distal convoluted tubule and negative values for the late distal convoluted tubule. Other studies (*Hayslett, Boulpaep,* and *Giebisch,* 1978; *Malnic* and *Giebisch,* 1972; *Wright,* 1971) have indi-

Table 5. Effect of Amiloride or Furosemide on Sodium Absorption and Potassium Secretion Across the Rabbit Distal Convoluted Tubule

Condition	Sodium Absorption	Potassium Secretion
Control	82.3 ± 18.2 (5)	9.3 ± 2.9 (5)
Amiloride (5 × 10^{-5} M)	31.8 ± 14.0 (5)	1.2 ± 0.8 (5)
Furosemide (5 × 10^{-5} M)	43.0 ± 9.7 (5)	13.3 ± 5.5 (5)

Values represent mean ±SEM (number of tubules). Drugs were placed in the perfusate.

DORSAL SURFACE

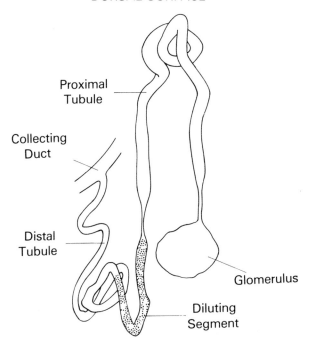

Fig. 1. Diagram of the amphibian nephron represents structure and orientation of nephrons found along the medial axis of the genital kidney. From *Stoner*, Am J Physiol 233:F438–F444, 1977.

cated that the potential difference in the early distal convoluted tubule is lower than that of the late distal nephron but still lumen-negative. Whether these differences are due to the species used or differences in technique is unknown at this time.

Studies of the transport capabilities of the amphibian distal convoluted tubule tend to reinforce the mammalian data just presented. The amphibian distal tubule has morphologically distinct segments similar to those of the rabbit. Unlike the rabbit, the amphibian distal tubule is of sufficient length that its early and late units can be studied separately *in vitro*. A schematic of the amphibian nephron is presented in Figure 1. This diagram applies to the nephron structure of the pelvic kidney of at least the frog and salamander. The term "diluting segment" denotes the early distal convoluted tubule. The term "distal tubule" is used here to indicate the late distal convoluted tubule.

Some transport properties of amphibian distal tubules are presented in Table 6. The early distal convoluted tubule (which we call the "diluting segment") transports substantial amounts of sodium and chloride out of the lumen and secretes some potassium into the lumen. While not shown in this table, the data for sodium and potassium transport are similar for the frog (*Rana pipiens*). In the salamander (*Ambystoma tigrinum*) the early distal tubule exhibited lumen-positive potential differences of about +14 mV. We have concluded from these data that its transport properties are similar to those of the thick ascending loop of Henle. The late distal tubule of the salamander transported sodium from the lumen to the bath and secreted potassium. These late segments had lumen-negative potential differences that averaged −29 mV. Sodium transport in the late portion of the amphibian nephron must be an active process, since it occurs against an electrochemical potential gradient.

The effect of amiloride on the transepithelial potential difference of these segments is shown in Table 7. Amiloride, 10^{-5} M, in the perfusate of the late distal nephron substantially reduced the lumen-negative potential difference. Ten times that concentration of the drug, placed on both sides of the early distal convoluted tubule, had no effect on the lumen-positive potential difference.

The effect of 10^{-5} M furosemide in the perfusate on the lumen-positive potential difference of the amphibian early distal tubule is also shown in Table 7. These data are qualitatively simlar to those I have presented for the distal convoluted tubule of the rabbit, and tend to reinforce our postulate that NaCl reabsorption in the distal convoluted tubule is the sum of at least two functionally distinct types of transport.

Recently *Morel, Chabardes*, and *Imbert* (1976) have presented biochemical evidence that the rabbit granular collecting duct is functionally distinct from the light portion of the cortical collecting tubule. Table 8 presents some data from three granular collecting tubules of the rabbit. The experimental protocol was similar to that used for the distal convoluted tubules except that the furosemide period was eliminated. As

Table 6. Characteristics of Ion Transport in Salamander Distal Nephron Segments

Nephron Segment	Spontaneous Voltage (mV)	Net ransport rate (pM mm^{-1} min^{-1})	
		Sodium Absorption	Potassium Secretion
Early Distal Tubule	+14.3 (5)	85.6 (5)	7.0 (5)
Late Distal Tubule	−39.4 (8)	21.2 (8)	2.3 (8)

Data modified from *Stoner* (1977).

Table 7.   Effect of Diuretics on the Spontaneous Voltage Across Amphibian Distal Nephron Segments

Nephron Segment	Voltage (mV)		
	Control*	Amiloride	Furosemide
Early Distal Tubule	+9.8	+9.8 $(10^{-4}$ M$)$	+1.0 $(10^{-5}$ M$)$
Late Distal Tubule	−26	−1.6 $(10^{-5}$ M$)$	—

* Represents mean of pre and postcontrol values.

Drugs were applied on the lumen surface. Values in parentheses indicate concentration of drug used. Data modified from *Stoner* (1977).

shown here, in the three tubules studied the potential difference was lumen-negative. Sodium was absorbed from and K secreted into the lumen. Amiloride, 10^{-5} M, inhibited all three of these transport processes to about 10% of their control values. It appears that the effect of amiloride in the granular cortical collecting tubule is similar to its effect on the light portion of the collecting tubule; however, I do not wish to imply that these segments have identical transport properties. We have recently demonstrated that the granular cortical collecting tubule has a parathyroid-sensitive calcium absorption mechanism, while the light cortical collecting tubule does not.

In conclusion, data have been presented which indicate that amiloride inhibits sodium transport and potassium secretion in at least three mammalian distal nephron segments: the distal convoluted tubule, the granular portion of the cortical collecting tubule and the light cortical collecting tubule. These data are consistent with the *in vivo* effects of the drug demonstrated with clearance and micropuncture techniques. At least in the light cortical collecting tubule, data indicate that the mechanism of action of amiloride is similar to that proposed in other epithelial tissues.

Table 8.   Effect of Amiloride on the Granular Cortical Collecting Tubule

	Control	Amiloride
Spontaneous Voltage (mV)	− 14.0 ± 1.7 (3)	−1.8 ± 0.5 (3)
Net Transport Rate, Lumen-to-bath (pM mm^{-1} min^{-1})		
Na$^+$	62.1 ± 16.7 (3)	7.0 ± 1.2 (3)
K$^+$	−6.2 ± 3.6 (3)	−0.4 ± 0.2 (3)

Values reported as mean ± SD (number of tubules).

REFERENCES

Baer, J.E., Jones, C.B., Spitzer, S.A., and Russo, H.F.   1967.   The potassium sparing and natriuretic activity of N-amidino-3,5-diamino-6-chloropyrazinecarboxamide hydrochloride dihydrate (amiloride hydrochloride). J Pharmacol Expl Therap 157:472–485

Barratt, L.J., Rector, F.C., Kokko, J.P., Tisher, C.C., and Seldin, D.W. 1975.   Transepithelial potential difference profile of the distal tubule of the rat kidney. Kidney Internat 8:368–375

Bentley, P.J.   1968.   Amiloride. A potent inhibitor of sodium transport across the toad bladder. J Physiol London 195:317–330

Bull, M.B., and Laragh, J.H.   1968.   Amiloride. A potassium-sparing natriuretic agent. Circulation 37:45–53

Burg, M.B., Grantham, J., Abramow, M., and Orloff, J.   1966.   Preparation and study of fragments of single rabbit nephrons. Am J Physiol 210:1293–1298

Burg, M., Stoner, L., Cardinal, J., and Green, N.   1973.   Furosemide effect on isolated perfused tubules. Am J Physiol 225:119–124

Burg, M., and Green, N.   1973.   Function of the thick ascending limb of Henle's loop. Am J Physiol 224:659–668

Dörge, A., and Nagel, W.   1970.   Effect of amiloride on Na transport in frog skin. II. Sodium transport pool and unidirectional fluxes. Arch Ges Physiol 321:91–101

Ehrlich, E.N., and Crabbé, J.   1968.   The mechanism of action of amipramizide. Arch Ges Physiol 302:79–96

Grantham, J.J., Burg, M.B., and Orloff, J.   1970.   The nature of transtubular sodium and potassium transport in isolated rabbit renal collecting tubule. J Clin Invest 49:1815–1826

Guignard, J.P., and Peters, G.   1970.   Effects of triamterene and amiloride on urinary acidification and potassium excretion in the rat. European J Pharmacol 10:255–267

Hayslett, J.P., Boulpaep, E.L., and Giebisch, G.H.   1978.   Factors influencing transepithelial potential difference in mammalian distal tubule. Am J Physiol Renal Fluid and Electrolyte 3:F182–F191

Malnic, G., and Giebisch, G.   1972.   Some electrical properties of distal tubular epithelium in the rat. Am J Physiol 223:797–808

Morel, F., Chabardes, D., and Imbert, M.   1976.   Functional segmentation of the rabbit distal tubule by microdetermination of hormone-dependent adenylate cyclase activity. Kidney Internat 9:264–277

O'Neil, R.G., and Helman, S.I.   1977.   Transport characteristics of renal collecting tubules: influences of DOCA and diet. Am J Physiol 233:F544–F558

Stoner, L.C.   1977.   Isolated perfused amphibian renal tubules. The diluting segment. Am J Physiol 233:F438–F444

Ussing, H.H.   1952.   Some aspects of the application of tracers in permeability studies. Advan Enzymol. 13:21–65.

Wright, F.S.   1971.   Increasing magnitude of electrical potential along the renal distal tubule. Am J Physiol 220:624–638

Effects of Amiloride on Sodium Fluxes in the Frog Skin

Thomas U. L. Biber

Department of Physiology
Medical College of Virginia
Richmond, Virginia 23298

The experiments reported here were done in collaboration with Drs. L.J. Cruz, T.L. Mullen and M.D. Wong (*Biber*, 1971, 1977; *Biber, Cruz,* and *Curran*, 1972; *Biber* and *Curran*, 1970; *Biber* and *Mullen*, 1976, 1977; *Biber* and *Sanders*, 1973; *Mullen* and *Biber*, 1978; *Wong* and *Biber*, 1974). The effect of amiloride on the isolated frog skin was tested by using two types of flux measurements: a) the unidirectional influx of Na across the outer border of the frog skin, and b) the unidirectional efflux of Na across the entire frog skin, from the serosal side to the external bathing medium.

Figure 1 shows a simplified model of the three compartments of frog skin. Compartments 1, 2 and 3 represent the outside bathing solution, the epithelial cells of frog skin and the serosal or inside bathing solution, respectively. The two types of flux determinations which were carried out can be labeled accordingly as J_{12}^{Na} (the influx of Na across the outer border of the epithelial cells from compartment 1 to compartment 2) and J_{31}^{Na} (the efflux of Na across the epithelial cells from compartment 3 to compartment 1).

We first became acquainted with amiloride in our laboratory when we studied the effect of rapid changes of Na concentration in the outside bathing solution on the epithelial potential and on the short-circuit current in frog skin (*Biber*, 1971). These experiments were carried out in the following way. Frog skin was mounted in a chamber which is schematically drawn on Figure 2. The frog skin is located in the middle chamber, with the outside surface facing downward. Appropriate connections permit the measurement of the transepithelial potential, and provisions are made for voltage clamping so that the short-circuit current can be recorded continuously. The solution bathing the outside surface of frog skin in the lower part of the chamber can be exchanged very rapidly.

61

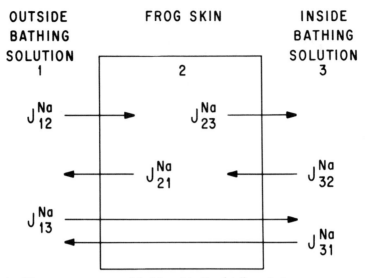

Fig. 1.   Three-compartment model of frog skin. For details see text.

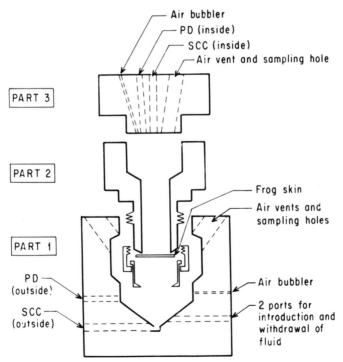

Fig. 2.   Chamber for determining the effects of rapid changes in Na and amiloride concentration in the outside bathing solution on short-circuit current and transepithelial potential. Chamber was also used for determination of $J_{12}{}^{Na}$. From *Biber* and *Curran*, J Gen Physiol 56:83–89, 1970.

Step changes in the concentration of about 40 mM were induced by injection of a concentrated NaCl solution into the outside bathing solution which contained a very low Na concentration of less than 1 mM. The time course of the transepithelial potential or of the short-circuit current was recorded on a storage oscilloscope.

As shown in Figure 3, a step change in the Na concentration of the outside bathing solution causes a rapid increase of the open-circuit transepithelial potential or the short-circuit current. Figure 4 shows the same effect (here labeled as control), i.e., an increase in current after a sudden addition of Na to the outside bathing solution. If a mixture of Na plus amiloride is added to the outside solution instead of only Na, after an initial increase in the current one observes an inhibition which sets in within about 20–50 msec. Such experiments provide an upper limit for the time within which amiloride acts on the short-circuit current. The actual time required is most likely even shorter, because amiloride may in fact reach the site of action later than Na due to differences in the diffusion coefficients for Na and for amiloride.

By far the greater part of the inhibition of the short-circuit current occurs within a very short time in an exponential fashion with a half-time in the range of 100 msec to a few seconds. However, one can regularly observe an additional, much slower inhibition with an exponential time course with a half-time in the range of several minutes. Such a dual time

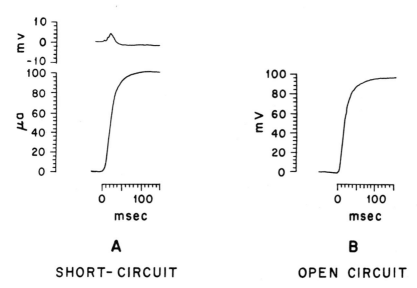

Fig. 3.   Effects of step changes in Na concentration in the outside bathing solution on short-circuit current measured in μa and on transepithelial potential measured in mV. The experiment was carried out under short-circuit as well as under open-circuit conditions, as indicated by panels A and B, respectively. From *Biber*, J Gen Physiol 58:131–144, 1971.

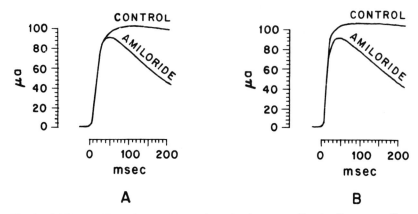

Fig. 4.   Inhibitory effect of amiloride on short-circuit current. For details see text. From *Biber*, J Gen Physiol 58:131–144, 1971.

course of action could be caused, for example, by different locations of the site of action in superficial and deeper cells or in different cell types, or by a secondary phenomenon connected with the exhaustion of the cellular Na transport pool.

The rapid onset of inhibition of the current after addition of amiloride and the reversibility of this effect after washing of the surface of the skin suggested that amiloride acts on frog skin by inhibiting the uptake of sodium from the outside bathing solution into the epithelial cells. For this reason, we proceeded to study the effect of amiloride on the unidirectional Na uptake or J_{12}^{Na}.

EFFECT OF AMILORIDE ON Na UPTAKE

Figure 5 illustrates the method used for the determination of the unidirectional Na influx across the outer surface of the frog skin. The isolated skin is mounted with the outside surface facing downward in a chamber which permits voltage clamping. Radioactive Na is added to the outside bathing solution, together with a labeled marker for extracellular spaces. After exposing the skin to the isotopes for a period of time, the skin is removed from the isotope-containing outside bathing solution, the serosal bathing solution is sucked out of the upper part of the chamber, and the outside surface is blotted to eliminate most of the remainder of the extracellularly located isotopes. Then, the skin is punched out of the chamber and dropped into $0.1N$ nitric acid. The determination of radioactive Na and extracellular markers in the eluate then permits the calculation of intracellular and extracellular sodium.

As can be seen from Figure 6, the uptake of radioactive Na is a linear function of time. This is what would be expected for this technique

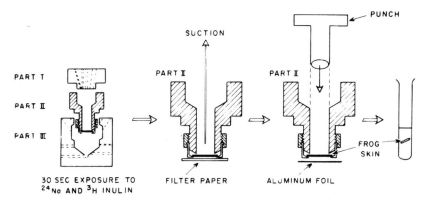

PART I

PART II

PART II

SUCTION

PUNCH

FROG SKIN

30 SEC EXPOSURE TO
^{24}Na AND ^{3}H INULIN

FILTER PAPER

ALUMINUM FOIL

Fig. 5. Schematic illustration of procedures for measuring Na uptake across the outside surface of frog skin. See text for details. From *Biber, T.U.L.* and *Sanders, M.L.* Influence of transepithelial potential difference on the sodium uptake at the outer surface of the isolated frog skin. J Gen Physiol 61:529–551, 1973.

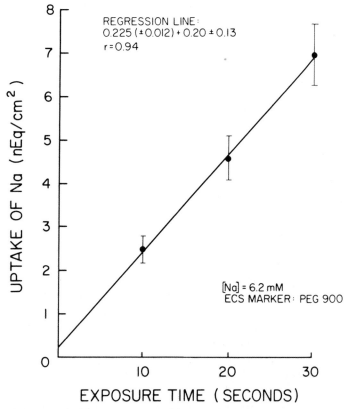

REGRESSION LINE:
0.225 (±0.012) + 0.20 ± 0.13
r = 0.94

[Na] = 6.2 mM
ECS MARKER: PEG 900

UPTAKE OF Na (nEq/cm²)

EXPOSURE TIME (SECONDS)

Fig. 6. Plot of Na uptake as measured by tissue accumulation of radioactive Na against time of exposure to the tracer in the outside bathing solution. From *Mullen* and *Biber*, Membrane Transport Processes, vol. 1, pp. 199–212, edited by J.F. Hoffman. Raven Press, New York, 1978.

of determining the initial rate of unidirectional uptake. The data shown here represent values which are corrected for the radioactive Na which remains after the blotting procedure on the outside surface of the skin. Initially, this correction for extracellular Na presented some problems. It was found that certain extracellular markers which were used for estimates of the extracellular space either did not distribute fast enough or completely throughout the entire extracellular space or they penetrated beyond the extracellular space (*Biber, Cruz*, and *Curran*, 1972). More recently, however, many different extracellular markers have been tested and remarkable agreement found between measurements carried out with different markers, provided that the precaution is taken of incubating the outside surface of the skin long enough if markers with a higher molecular weight are used (*Mullen* and *Biber*, 1978). Polyethylene glycol 900 or PEG 900 and K^{42} were particularly suitable for these measurements. Recent experiments in which we used either PEG 900 and/or K^{42} as extracellular markers confirmed the most important conclusions drawn from earlier experiments. The linear uptake shown in Figure 6 was obtained with PEG 900 as extracellular marker.

One of the major factors in evaluating the effect of amiloride on Na uptake was the observation that the Na uptake is closely related to the short-circuit current. Figure 7 shows the relationship between short-circuit current and Na uptake measured with PEG 900 as extracellular marker. The determinations were made either at a Na concentration of 6 mM (as shown on the left of Fig. 7) or at a sodium concentration of 100 mM (as shown on the right). From such a plot of Na uptake against the short-circuit current it can be seen that the Na uptake varies exactly in proportion to the short-circuit current. In Figure 8 essentially the same relationship can be seen when K^{42} is used as an extracellular marker. K^{42} can be used for this purpose because the outside surface of the skin has a very low potassium permeability.

Figure 9 shows the results of Na uptake measurements carried out at different Na concentrations. Such results indicate that the Na uptake saturates with increasing Na concentration and that the Na uptake and the short-circuit current are practically identical over the entire range. The insert demonstrates that the points for both the Na uptake and the short-circuit give a close fit to a line when plotted as flux against flux divided by concentration. There is good evidence from autoradiographic studies carried out in our laboratory (*Wong* and *Biber*, 1974 and unpublished results) and from X-ray microanalysis carried out by Dörge and collaborators (*Dörge*, 1978) that the Na uptake determined with this method actually measures the undirectional influx of Na from the outside bathing solution into the outermost-located (first) living cell layer. Thus, the Na uptake across the outwardfacing cell membrane of the epithelial cells is practically equal to the short-circuit current.

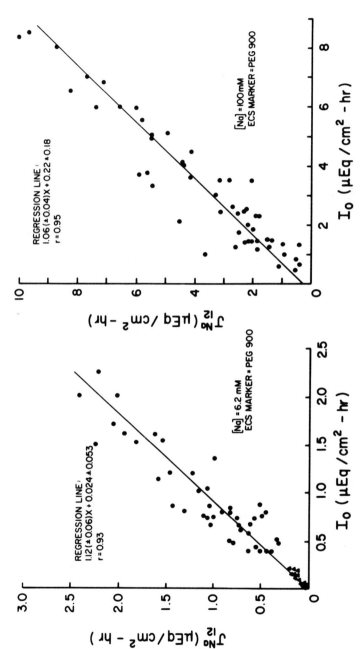

Fig. 7. Na uptake plotted against short-circuit current. Na concentration of the bath was 6.2 mM on the left and 100 mM on the right. PEG 900 was used as extracellular marker. From *Mullen* and *Biber*, Membrane Transport Processes, vol. I, pp. 199–212, edited by J.F. Hoffman. Raven Press, New York, 1978.

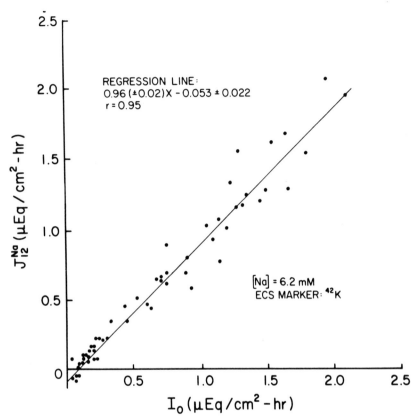

Fig. 8. Na uptake plotted against short-circuit current. Na concentration was 6.2 mM. K⁴² was used as extracellular marker. From *Mullen* and *Biber*, Membrane Transport Processes, vol. 1, pp. 199–212, edited by J.F. Hoffman. Raven Press, New York, 1978.

Another plot of Na uptake vs short-circuit current is shown in Figure 10. The triangles represent Na uptake values which were obtained after application of amiloride (*Biber*, 1977). The location of these points indicates that 10^{-5} M amiloride inhibits both the short-circuit current and Na uptake by the same amount. These experiments were carried out at a Na concentration of 6 mM, but an equivalent reduction of the Na uptake and the short-circuit current was also obtained at a Na concentration of 100 mM after amiloride treatment. The data plotted on Figure 11 indicate that the results are virtually identical, regardless of whether the skin is preincubated in the amiloride for 12 min or the amiloride is added simultaneously with radioactive Na for a time space of 30 sec. The data shown in this figure were obtained in initial studies (*Biber*, 1971) and therefore include an overestimate of the Na uptake by about 0.45 μEq hr^{-1} cm^{-2} due to incomplete correction of the extracellular space.

EFFECT OF AMILORIDE ON Na EFFLUX

The effect of amiloride on the Na efflux across the frog skin, i.e., the flux from the serosal bathing solution into the outside bathing solution or J_{31}^{Na}, was recently tested (*Biber* and *Mullen*, 1976, 1977). Figure 12 depicts a diagram of the chambers used to measure the Na efflux across the frog skin. The chamber is designed to minimize the effect of edge-damage by using soft gaskets and by exerting only a minimal pressure to prevent the bathing solutions from leaking out of the chamber. The pressure is actually less than the pressure exerted by the frog's own weight when the frog rests on the belly. To our great surprise, it was dis-covered that the Na efflux measured in such chambers exhibits saturation kinetics (*Biber* and *Mullen*, 1976). This can be seen in Figure 13 on a plot of Na efflux against Na concentration, or on the plot of flux against flux over concentration shown in the insert. The Na efflux measured in such chambers is low, with a V_{max} of 32 μEq hr^{-1} cm^{-2} and an apparent K_m of 4 mM.

On the other hand, it was found that the efflux of nonelectrolytes such as PEG$_{900}$, sucrose or mannitol is a linear function of the concentra-

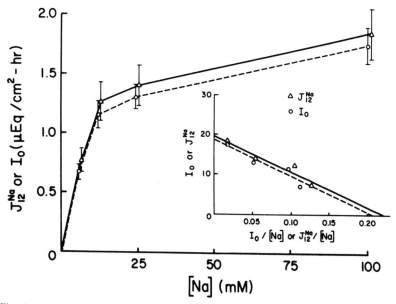

Fig. 9. Plot of Na uptake against Na concentration (large plot) or against Na uptake divided by Na concentration (insert). Triangles indicate data for Na uptake. The cor-responding plots for the short-circuit current (I_0) are marked by circles. From *Mullen* and *Biber*, Membrane Transport Processes, vol. 1, pp. 199–212, edited by J.F. Hoffman. Raven Press, New York, 1978.

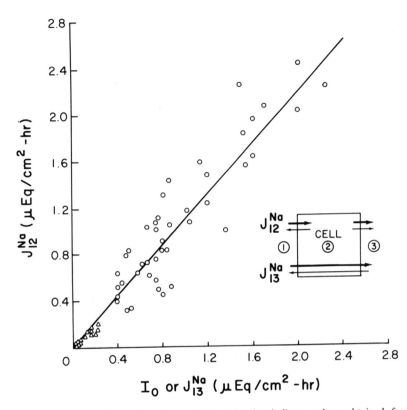

Fig. 10.   Plot of $J_{12}{}^{Na}$ against I_0 or $J_{13}{}^{Na}$. Triangles indicate values obtained from amiloride-treated skins; circles are control values. From *Biber*, Diuretics in Research and Clinics, pp. 58–63, edited by W. Siegenthaler, R. Beckerhoff and N. Vetter. Georg Thieme Publishers, Stuttgart, 1977.

tion. This suggests that the nonelectrolyte fluxes proceed via paracellular shunt-pathways, a notion which is strongly supported by autoradiographic studies carried out in our laboratory in which it could be observed that mannitol is selectively restricted to intercellular spaces throughout the entire frog skin under a wide variety of conditions (*Biber* and *Wong*, unpublished data).

Figure 14 shows an example for the large increase in Na efflux observed after treatment with ouabain. Despite large changes in Na efflux after ouabain treatment, a saturation of the Na efflux can still be observed. As Figure 15 shows, the V_{max} increased to some 167 μEq hr^{-1} cm^{-2} and the apparent Michaelis constant increased from 4 mM under control conditions to 5.6 mM after ouabain treatment. It should be mentioned here that, although the Na efflux increases after application of ouabain, there was no significant change in nonelectrolyte fluxes after ouabain treatment. Hence, the Na efflux differs from the nonelectrolyte effluxes not only by exhibiting saturation under control conditions but also in the response to ouabain. All this can be taken to suggest that the Na efflux proceeds via a transcellular pathway rather than via an extracellular shunt-pathway.

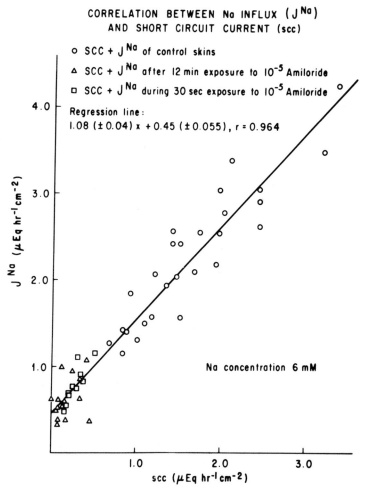

Fig. 11.   Plot of Na uptake against short-circuit current. For details see text. From *Biber*, J Gen Physiol 58:131–144, 1971.

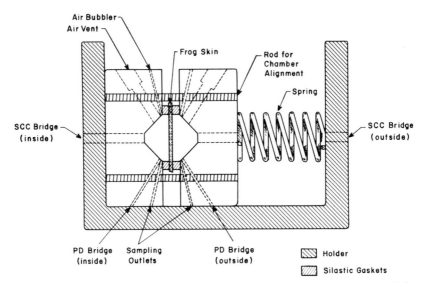

Fig. 12. Schematic drawing of chamber used for Na-efflux measurements. From *Biber* and *Mullen*, Am J Physiol 232(1):C67–C75, 1977.

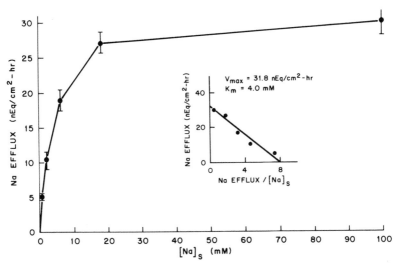

Fig. 13. Plot of Na efflux against the Na concentration (large plot) or against the Na efflux divided by the Na concentration (insert). From *Biber* and *Mullen*, Am J Physiol 231:995–1001, 1976.

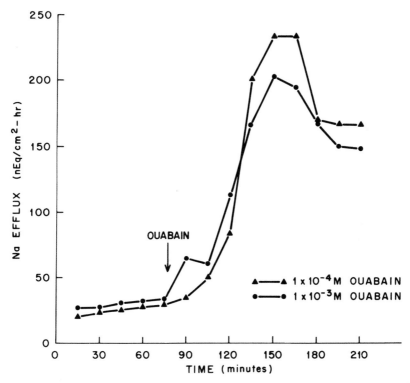

Fig. 14. Effect of ouabain on Na efflux. From *Biber* and *Mullen*, Am J Physiol 232(1):C67–C75, 1977.

The effect of amiloride on the Na efflux is shown in Figure 16. These experiments were carried out at a Na concentration of 6 mM. The Na efflux decreased after application of amiloride. The decrease due to amiloride was more pronounced when the skins were pretreated with ouabain. From Figure 17 it becomes clear that the ratio of nonelectrolyte permeability to Na permeability changes after application of amiloride. Since the permeability to nonelectrolytes (mannitol was used here) remains unchanged after amiloride, we can say that the Na permeability decreases substantially, to about one-sixth, when measured at a Na concentration of 6 mM, and that the Na permeability increases to about three times the control value when measured at a Na concentration of 100 mM. Treatment with amiloride may cause an even greater inhibition of Na efflux than shown here, up to 95% at low Na concentrations. Figure 18 represents a plot of the Na efflux determined in amiloride-treated skins against the Na concentration. Obviously, treatment with

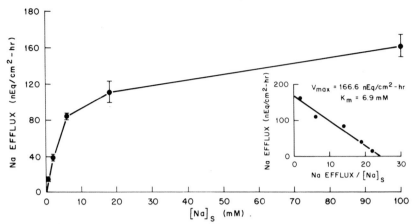

Fig. 15. Na efflux values obtained in ouabain-treated skins. The data are plotted as in Figure 13. From *Biber* and *Mullen*, Am J Physiol 231:995–1001, 1976.

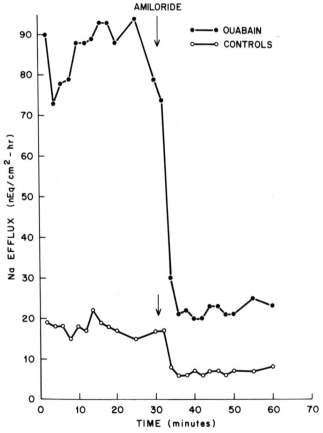

Fig. 16. Effect of amiloride on Na efflux. From *Biber* and *Mullen*, Am J Physiol 232(1):C67–C75, 1977.

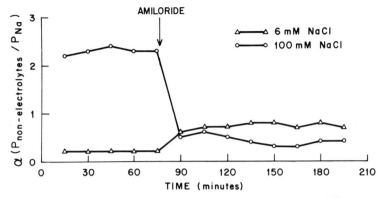

Fig. 17. Effect of amiloride on α, the ratio of nonelectrolyte permeability over Na   016
permeability. From *Biber* and *Mullen*, Am J Physiol 232(1):C67–C75, 1977.

amiloride eliminates the saturation phenomenon for the Na efflux. The
effect of amiloride on the Na efflux was measured in ouabain-treated
skins and in skins which were not exposed to ouabain. Ouabain treatment
increases the Na efflux by a factor of about three.

Amiloride is not the only compound which causes elimination of the
saturation phenomenon for Na efflux. Treatment with 10^{-4} molar
dinitrophenol results in a very large Na efflux, as can be seen on Figure
19. The Na efflux increased from about 35 μEq cm^{-2} hr^{-1} to over 800

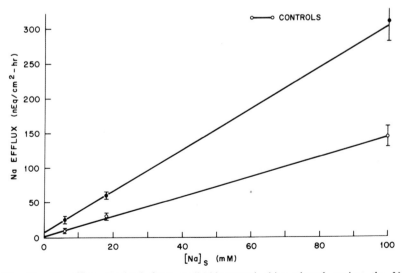

Fig. 18. Na efflux obtained from amiloride-treated skins plotted against the Na
concentration. Solid circles indicate Na efflux from skins which, in addition to amiloride,
were also exposed to ouabain. From *Biber* and *Mullen*, Am J Physiol 231:995–1001, 1976.

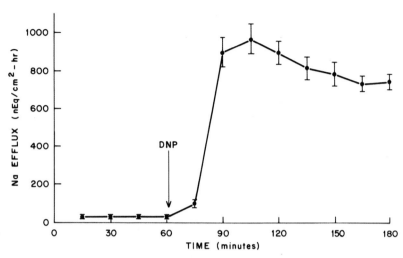

Fig. 19.   Effect of dinitrophenol (DNP) on Na efflux. From *Biber* and *Mullen*, Am J Physiol 232(1):C67–C75, 1977.

μEq cm^{-2} hr^{-1}. Again, the nonelectrolyte permeability remained unchanged. Figure 20 demonstrates that, in addition, DNP also abolishes the saturation phenomenon for Na efflux.

In summary, amiloride not only blocks the entry of sodium across the outward-facing cell membrane of the epithelial cells but also causes substantial changes in sodium efflux, which seems to proceed transcellularly across the epithelial cells. The elimination of the saturation

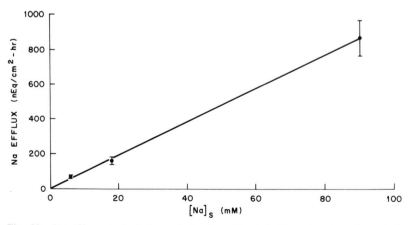

Fig. 20.   Na efflux obtained from dinitrophenol-treated skins plotted against the Na concentration. From *Biber* and *Mullen*, Am J Physiol 231:995–1001, 1976.

phenomenon after amiloride treatment raises the question of whether the outward-facing cell membrane of the outermost living cell layer is involved in the saturation phenomenon for the sodium efflux.

REFERENCES

Biber, T.U.L. 1971. Effect of changes in transepithelial transport on the uptake of sodium across the outer surface of frog skin. J Gen Physiol 58:131–144

Biber, T.U.L. 1977. Uptake of sodium in epithelia. Effect of amiloride. In *Diuretics in research and clinics*, eds. W. Siegenthaler, R. Beckerhoff and W. Vetter, pp. 58–63. Stuttgart: George Thieme Publishers

Biber, T.U.L., Cruz, L.J., and Curran, P.E. 1972. Sodium influx at the outer surface of frog skin. Evaluation of different extracellular markers. J Membrane Biol 7:365–376

Biber, T.U.L., and Curran, P.F. 1970. Direct measurement of uptake of sodium at the outer surface of the frog skin. J Gen Physiol 56:83–89

Biber, T.U.L., and Mullen, T.L. 1976. Saturation kinetics of sodium efflux across isolated frog skin. Am J Physiol 231:995–1001

Biber, T.U.L., and Mullen, T.L. 1977. Effect of inhibitors on transepithelial efflux of Na and nonelectrolytes in frog skin. Am J Physiol 232(1):C67–C75

Biber, T.U.L., and Sanders, M.L. 1973. Influence of transepithelial potential difference on sodium uptake at the outer surface of the frog skin. J Gen Physiol 61:529–551

Dörge, A. 1978. An x-ray microanalysis of cellular electrolytes in frog skin epithelia: The site of action of amiloride and the pathway of Na^+. This symposium

Mullen, T.L., and Biber, T.U.L. 1978. Sodium uptake across outer surface of the frog skin. In *Membrane transport processes*, volume 1 ed. J.E. Hoffman, pp. 199–212. New York: Raven Press

Wong, M.D., and Biber, T.U.L. 1974. Location of Na-transport steps in isolated frog skin. Fed Proc 33:215

Effects of Amiloride on Transepithelial Sodium Transport and Glucose Metabolism in Toad Bladder

*Geoffrey W. G. Sharp**

Biochemical Pharmacology Unit
Massachusetts General Hospital
Boston, Massachusetts 02114

INTRODUCTION

Early studies on transporting epithelia demonstrated that when amiloride was applied to the outside of amphibian skin or the apical surface of the toad bladder, active sodium transport was blocked by a rapid and easily reversible mechanism (*Baba et al.*, 1968; *Bentley*, 1968; *Ehrlich* and *Crabbé*, 1968; *Eigler, Kelter,* and *Renner*, 1967). Amiloride, at comparable concentration, had no effect on sodium transport when applied to the inside of the skin or the serosal surface of the bladder. Thus, the evidence suggested a direct interaction of amiloride with a component of the membrane associated with the entry of sodium into the transport pathway. The interaction is external to the cell and amiloride does not accumulate in the tissue from the apical side (*Robbie*, 1971). As amiloride acts on sites of sodium transport which are affected by aldosterone and as it reverses the effects of aldosterone, the interaction of these two agents has been studied with respect to both transport and glucose metabolism. It was anticipated that amiloride would act to deprive the transport pathway of sodium, and that the tissue response would be similar to that observed when Na^+-free media are used on the apical surface. However, a potentially important difference between the effect of

This work was supported in part by grants from the John A. Hartford Foundation, Inc. and the Public Health Service, research grants HE-06664 from the National Heart Institute and AM-04501 from the National Institute of Arthritis and Metabolic Disease.

* Present address: Department of Physiology, Tufts University School of Medicine, Boston, Massachusetts 02111

amiloride and the effect of Na$^+$-free media was detected, i.e., amiloride could affect the hexose monophosphate shunt pathway and reverse the inhibitory effect of aldosterone on this alternate pathway of glucose metabolism. Thus, this paper will consider: a) the effect of aldosterone to inhibit the activity of the hexose monophosphate shunt pathway and its relation to sodium transport; b) the validity of the methods used to estimate the hexose monophosphate shunt pathway; and c) the effects of amiloride on the shunt pathway.

The results suggest that the hexose monophosphate shunt pathway can be controlled by a component of the apical membrane which is affected by aldosterone, and by amiloride. Remarkably, the effect of amiloride is exerted from the exterior of the transporting cells.

METHODS

Full details of the methods used have been published previously for Na$^+$ transport (*Sharp* and *Leaf*, 1964, 1965), the measurement of $^{14}CO_2$ evolution from [1-^{14}C], [2-^{14}C] and [6-^{14}C] glucose (*Kirchberger et al.*, 1968; *Kirchberger, Chen,* and *Sharp,* 1971; *Beckman et al.,* 1974) the pathway separation (*Kirchberger et al.,* 1971; *Wood, Katz,* and *Landau,* 1963) and ^{14}C-amiloride accumulation studies (*Robbie,* 1971).

^{14}C-Glucose was obtained from New England Nuclear Corporation, Boston, MA. Purity was greater than 99% and was checked by thin-layer silica-gel chromatography in an ethyl acetate-isopropanol-water solvent system (130:75:30 by vol) followed by radioautography.

Nonradioactive amiloride hydrochloride dihydrate (MK 870) and ^{14}C-amiloride (167 μCi/mg, labeled at the guanidinyl carbon), prepared by Dr. C. Rosenblum, were the gift of Dr. John Baer of Merck, Sharp, and Dohme. Aldosterone was kindly provided by Dr. M.M. Pechet of the Research Institute for Medicine and Chemistry, Cambridge, MA. Spirolactone SC 14266 was a gift from G.D. Searle and Company.

RESULTS AND DISCUSSION

Inhibition of the Hexosemonophosphate Shunt Pathway by Aldosterone

$^{14}CO_2$ Evolution from [1-^{14}C] and [6-^{14}C]Glucose

The basis for the use of [1-^{14}C] and [6-^{14}C]glucose as a method for the study of glucose metabolism by the Embden-Meyerhof pathway and the hexose monophosphate shunt pathway is shown in Figure 1. In this figure the fate of ^{14}C in positions 1 and 6 of glucose (indicated by the triangle and circle, respectively) is shown. It can be seen that the carbon

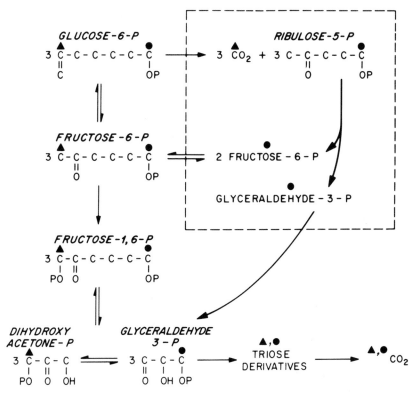

Fig. 1. $^{14}CO_2$ evolution from [1-^{14}C] and [6-^{14}C]-labeled glucose during metabolism via the Embden-Meyerhof and hexose monophosphate shunt pathways. [1-^{14}C] is indicated by the triangle and [6-^{14}C] by the closed circle.

atoms in the 1 and 6 positions of glucose are handled similarly by the Embden-Meyerhof pathway and contribute equally to $^{14}CO_2$ evolution. In the hexosemonophosphate shunt pathway only the 1 carbon is converted to CO_2. Thus, [1-^{14}C]glucose metabolized by the shunt pathway will liberate all its [1-^{14}C] as $^{14}CO_2$. [6-^{14}C]glucose will not liberate $^{14}CO_2$ in this pathway. Consequently, an estimate of hexose monophosphate shunt pathway activity can be obtained by subtracting the $^{14}CO_2$ evolved with [6-^{14}C]glucose from that evolved with [1-^{14}C]glucose.

This method is liable to error in that it assumes that the Embden-Meyerhof and hexosemonophosphate shunt pathways are the only pathways of glucose metabolism, that no changes in recycling occur and that there is complete equilibration between fructose-6-P and glucose-6-P. It is, however, a useful indicator of changed activity in the shunt pathway, particularly when the changes in $^{14}CO_2$ evolution are large. This is the case for aldosterone. When toad bladders were incubated for 15 hr in the presence or absence of 4×10^{-7} M aldosterone, the hormone resulted in a 200% increase in $^{14}CO_2$ evolution from [6-^{14}C]glucose, a 30% decrease in $^{14}CO_2$ evolution from [1-^{14}C]glucose and a 90% decrease in $^{14}CO_2$ evolution from [1-^{14}C] minus [6-^{14}C]glucose (*Kirchberger et al.*, 1968). That this is a primary effect of aldosterone and not dependent upon increased sodium transport or the energy cost of transport was shown by performing the experiments in the absence of Na^+ in the mucosal medium. Under these conditions, with no change in the evolution of $^{14}CO_2$ from [6-^{14}C]glucose, aldosterone caused a significant inhibition of $^{14}CO_2$ evolution from [1-^{14}C]glucose (*Kirchberger et al.*, 1968).

Pathway Separation by Lactate Labeling

Because of the primary nature of this effect of aldosterone and because it could help shed light on the stimulation of sodium transport, further tests were performed to document that the effect was in fact an inhibition of the shunt pathway. Thus, the method of *Wood, Katz,* and *Landau* (1963) was used to estimate the extent of the pathway in toad bladder and the effect of aldosterone. The method is based on the following formulation of the hexose monophosphate shunt:

3 glucose-6-P $\rightarrow$ 3 CO_2 + 3 pentose-P
3 pentose-P $\rightarrow$ 2 fructose-6-P + 1 glyceraldehyde-3-P
2 fructose-6-P $\rightarrow$ 2 glucose-6-P
1 glucose-6-P $\rightarrow$ CO_2 + 1 glyceraldehyde-3-P

This model assumes complete recycling of fructose-6-P to glucose-6-P. This recycling will dilute the specific activity of the labeled glucose-6-P when [1-^{14}C]glucose, but not [6-^{14}C]glucose, is the substrate because of the loss of $^{14}CO_2$ via the pentose cycle. When the hexosemonophosphate shunt pathway and the Embden-Meyerhof pathway are the sole pathways of glucose metabolism, it can be shown that the dilution factor, called

$$Q, = \frac{1}{1 + 2HMP}.$$

As the trioses and derivatives (e.g., lactate) are labeled by [1-^{14}C]glucose only via the EM pathway and by [6-^{14}C]glucose via both the Em and HMP pathways, the ratio of the triose labeling may be derived as follows:

$$\frac{1-^{14}C}{6-^{14}C} = \frac{EM \times Q}{EM + HMP}$$

but EM = 1 − HMP

$$\frac{1-^{14}C}{6-^{14}C} = \frac{1 - HMP \times Q}{1}$$

substituting $\dfrac{1}{1 + 2\,\mathrm{HMP}}$ for Q

$$\dfrac{1\text{-}^{14}\mathrm{C}\text{ in triose}}{6\text{-}^{14}\mathrm{C}\text{ in triose}} = \dfrac{1 - \mathrm{HMP}}{1 + 2\mathrm{HMP}}$$

Bearing in mind the assumptions underlying this method, the extent of the hexose monophosphate shunt pathway to glucose metabolism can be determined. This was done by purifying the lactate produced by toad bladder in the presence and absence of aldosterone, determining its specific activity when incubated with [1-^{14}C]glucose and with [6-^{14}C]glucose and calculating the percentage contribution of the shunt to glucose metabolism. In nine control bladders it was calculated that the shunt pathway was responsible for 23% of the glucose metabolized. In contrast, after treatment with aldosterone for 6 hr (16 hr in one case), the shunt pathway was inhibited to the extent that it contributed only 7% of the glucose metabolized. The magnitude of this change makes it highly unlikely that some other pathway of glucose metabolism could be involved.

Assessment of Recycling by $^{14}CO_2$ Evolution from [2-^{14}C]Glucose

The pathway separation described above ($^{14}CO_2$ evolution from [1-^{14}C] and [6-^{14}C]glucose) assumes complete recycling. If recycling were not complete, then one means of decreasing $^{14}CO_2$ from [1-^{14}C] − [6-^{14}C]glucose would be to increase the extent of recycling. This has the effect of decreasing the specific activity of the glucose 6-phosphate pool by removing the ^{14}C from [1-^{14}C]glucose and returning unlabeled glucose-6-phosphate via fructose 6-phosphate. As an increase in recycling can be detected by a decrease in $^{14}CO_2$ from [2-^{14}C] − [6-^{14}C]glucose, the effect of aldosterone on the evolution of $^{14}CO_2$ from [1-^{14}C], [2-^{14}C] and [6-^{14}C] glucose was measured (*Kirchberger et al.*, 1971). $^{14}CO_2$ from [2-^{14}C] glucose is released in the hexosemonophosphate shunt pathway only after the molecule has passed down the pathway, has the unlabeled carbon removed from the 1 position and recycles to glucose 6-phosphate so that the original 2-^{14}C is now in the 1 position. This radioactive carbon is removed during the second passage through the cycle (i.e., after recycling). The results showed that $^{14}CO_2$ evolution from [2-^{14}C] minus [6-^{14}C] glucose was significantly decreased (control bladders 0.35 μmoles glucose/g dry wt/hr; aldosterone-treated 0.03 μmoles/g dry wt/hr, $\Delta = 0.32 \pm 0.11$, n = 10, P < 0.02). Thus, it was concluded that recycling does occur to a large extent and that, because the [2-^{14}C] minus [6-^{14}C] parameter decreased, the hexose monophosphate shunt pathway is inhibited by aldosterone. Furthermore, it can be concluded that the use of $^{14}CO_2$ measurements from [1-^{14}C] minus [6-^{14}C]glucose is a convenient and simple indicator of the effect of aldosterone on the hexose monophosphate shunt pathway.

The Mineralocorticoid Nature of the Inhibition
of the Hexose Monophosphate Shunt Pathway by Aldosterone

Having determined that the effect of aldosterone to decrease $^{14}CO_2$ evolution from [1-^{14}C] minus [6-^{14}C]glucose is the result of an inhibition of the hexose monophosphate shunt pathway, it was necessary to determine whether the effect was mineralocorticoid (i.e., related to the stimulation of sodium transport), due to the glucocorticoid potential of aldosterone or a nonspecific steroid effect. Several tests were performed.

Time Course Studies

One characteristic of the response of sodium transport to aldosterone is the latent period between addition of hormone and onset of increased sodium transport. Generally, this latent period is at least 1 hr, after which a steady increase in the rate of sodium transport occurs. It was found that the $^{14}CO_2$ evolution from [1-^{14}C] minus [6-^{14}C]glucose bore an inverse relationship to the rate of sodium transport after stimulation by aldosterone (*Kirchberger et al.*, 1968).

Dose Response Characteristics

The bladder responds to aldosterone from concentrations of approximately 10^{-9} - 10^{-7} M with a graded increase in sodium transport. The effect on glucose metabolism of increasing concentration of aldosterone was therefore examined. It was found that changes in the hexose-monophosphate shunt pathway occurred over the same concentration range which caused minimal to maximum effects on sodium transport (*Kirchberger et al.*, 1968).

Inhibition by Actinomycin D

Actinomycin D blocks the stimulation of sodium transport by aldosterone. Its effect on the aldosterone-induced change in glucose metabolism was therefore examined. In experiments performed in the absence of sodium in the mucosal medium to prevent changes in [6-^{14}C] glucose utilization, actinomycin D abolished the effect of aldosterone to decrease $^{14}CO_2$ from [1-^{14}C]glucose (*Kirchberger et al.*, 1968).

Steroid Specificity

To examine the specificity of the steroidal effect on the metabolism of glucose, the effects of dexamethasone, deoxycorticosterone, progesterone and cortisone on sodium transport and glucose metabolism were tested. Dexamethasone and deoxycorticosterone (5×10^{-7} M) reduced $^{14}CO_2$ from, [1-^{14}C] minus [6-^{14}C]glucose, whereas progesterone at the same concentration failed to affect glucose metabolism. Other experiments showed that dexamethasone stimulates sodium transport in this tissue even at concentrations as low as 10^{-9} M, whereas progesterone has no effect on sodium transport at the concentration studied here. Cortisone, like progesterone, had no effect upon either sodium transport or glucose metabolism. Thus, the changes in glucose metabolism correlated with the presence of a hormonal effect on sodium transport.

Further studies examined the relative potencies of known mineralocorticoids (aldosterone and deoxycorticosterone) with a glucocorticoid (cortisol) under paired conditions. A low concentration of these steroids (5×10^{-9} M) was tested. Under these conditions $^{14}CO_2$ evolution from 6-^{14}C glucose was significantly increased by aldosterone and deoxycorticosterone but not by cortisol. Similarly, the $^{14}CO_2$ evolution from [1-^{14}C] – [6-^{14}C] glucose was significantly decreased by aldosterone and deoxycorticosterone but not by cortisol. Therefore, it appears with respect to the inhibition of $^{14}CO_2$ release from [1-^{14}C] – [6-^{14}C]glucose that the two potent mineralocorticoids, aldosterone and deoxycorticosterone, are more effective than cortisol (*Kirchberger et al.*, 1971).

Inhibition by a Specific
Mineralocorticoid Antagonist Spirolactone SC14266

Before studying the effect of SC14266 (a water-soluble spirolactone) to antagonize the effects of aldosterone, control experiments were performed to determine the highest concentration of SC14266 which could be used. In these control experiments 10^{-4} M spirolactone SC 14266 significantly decreased the $^{14}CO_2$ evolution from [1-^{14}C]glucose and also decreased, though not significantly, the $^{14}CO_2$ evolution from [6-^{14}C]glucose. At this concentration an immediate and nonspecific inhibition of sodium transport is also observed. At 10^{-5} M spirolactone SC 14266 a nonsignificant decrease of $^{14}CO_2$ evolution occurred, while at 10^{-6} M no effect of spirolactone SC 14266 upon glucose metabolism was detectable (*Kirchberger et al.*, 1971). Consequently, concentrations of spirolactone SC 14266 between 10^{-6} and 10^{-5} M were used for the antagonism studies. These concentrations, however, restrict the concentration of aldosterone which may be used because of the need to maintain a spirolactone excess of at least 1000-fold that of the hormone.

Effects of Spirolactone SC 14266 (2.5×10^{-6} M
and 5.0×10^{-6} M) and Aldosterone (2.5×10^{-9} M) upon
$^{14}CO_2$ Release from [1-^{14}C] – [6-^{14}C]Glucose

SC 14266 at 2.5×10^{-6} M had no effect upon the $^{14}CO_2$ evolution from either [1-^{14}C] or [6-^{14}C]glucose. Aldosterone produced its typical effects with an 83% increase in the $^{14}CO_2$ from [6-^{14}C] glucose and a 46% decrease in the [1-^{14}C] – [6-^{14}C] parameter. When the tissue was subjected to both aldosterone and spirolactone, the effect of the hormone was inhibited and no longer significantly different from control values. Thus, a 1000-fold excess of spirolactone SC 14266 inhibited, though not completely, both the increase in $^{14}CO_2$ from [6-^{14}C]glucose and the decrease in the [1-^{14}C] – [6-^{14}C] parameter. In the second series of experiments performed with a 2000-fold excess of spirolactone SC 14266, inhibition of the effect of aldosterone upon [1-^{14}C] – [6-^{14}C] glucose utilization was almost complete. Spirolactone SC 14266 at these concentrations had no effect in the absence of aldosterone.

Effects of Spirolactone SC 14266 (5×10^{-6} M) and Dexamethasone (2.5×10^{-9} M) upon $^{14}CO_2$ Release from [1-^{14}C] and [6-^{14}C]Glucose

Dexamethasone caused a significant increase in $^{14}CO_2$ from [6-^{14}C] glucose and a significant decrease in $^{14}CO_2$ from [1-^{14}C] – [6-^{14}C]glucose. Spirolactone inhibited both these effects. Thus, the mineralocorticoid antagonist blocks the rise in sodium transport and the inhibition of the pentose cycle due to aldosterone and dexamethasone.

It is concluded that the effect of aldosterone on the hexose-monophosphate shunt pathway is "mineralocorticoid" in character and is not secondary to changed rates of sodium transport. Therefore, it is possible that the changed activity of the shunt pathway could be related to the mechanism by which aldosterone stimulates sodium transport.

Effects of Amiloride on Sodium Transport

Figure 2 shows the effects of three concentrations of amiloride on sodium transport. When amiloride was applied to the mucosal surface of the bladders, Na^+ transport was rapidly and markedly inhibited. The inhibition was 69% at 10^{-6} M, 85% at 10^{-5} M and 89% at 10^{-4} M. In contrast, the effects from the serosal side were slight and gradual. No inhibition of Na^+ transport was observed at 10^{-6} or 10^{-5} M, while at 10^{-4} M an inhibition of only 15% was observed. This inhibition of transport was different in character from that observed when amiloride was added to the mucosal surface. In the latter situation the inhibition of transport is extremely rapid and most of the inhibition occurs within the first minute after application. In contrast, serosal addition of the amiloride results in a slow and progressive decrease in transport.

Effects of Amiloride on Glucose Metabolism

In preliminary experiments paired pieces of toad bladders were incubated for 5 hr in the presence or absence of aldosterone. Amiloride (1×10^{-6} M) was then added where appropriate so that $^{14}CO_2$ evolution from

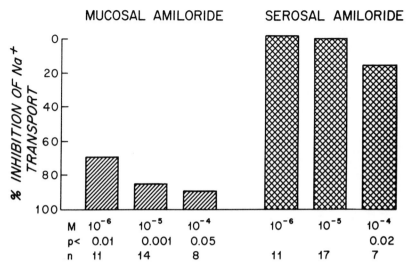

Fig. 2.   Inhibition of sodium transport by different concentrations of amiloride applied to either the mucosal or the serosal side of the toad bladder. Results expressed as percent inhibition relative to untreated control tissues.

[1-^{14}C]glucose and [6-^{14}C]glucose could be measured under four sets of conditions: control conditions, in the presence of amiloride, and after aldosterone treatment in the presence and absence of amiloride. The incubations were performed in flasks in the conventional manner so that amiloride bathed both the serosal and mucosal surfaces of the tissue.

Under these conditions amiloride significantly inhibited $^{14}CO_2$ evolution from [6-^{14}C]glucose, in the presence or absence of aldosterone. Aldosterone significantly increased $^{14}CO_2$ from [6-^{14}C]glucose, while exerting its usual inhibitory effect upon the hexose monophosphate shunt pathway ([1-^{14}C] − [6-^{14}C]) as seen by a change from 0.72 μmoles/g dry wt/hr under control conditions to 0.32 after treatment with aldosterone. Amiloride was found to partially reverse the inhibition induced by aldosterone, $^{14}CO_2$ evolution increasing from 0.32 to 0.59 μmoles/g dry wt/hr. No significant increase was detected in control tissue treated with amiloride.

With the demonstration of an inverse relationship between sodium transport and the hexose monophosphate shunt pathway, as evidenced by stimulation of the shunt pathway with amiloride in the presence of aldosterone, it became important to define the amiloride effect. Thus, the effect of either mucosal or serosal application was studied. These results are presented in Figures 3 and 4. When applied to the mucosal surface only, amiloride inhibited the evolution of $^{14}CO_2$ from [6-^{14}C]glucose. This presumably reflects the inhibition of sodium transport and reduced energy requirements. More importantly, a reversal of the aldosterone-induced inhibition of the hexose monophosphate shunt pathway was observed (see Fig. 3). In contrast, when applied to the serosal side, amiloride had no effect on $^{14}CO_2$ evolution from [1-^{14}C] minus [6-^{14}C]glucose, although a slight but significant decrease in $^{14}CO_2$ from [6-^{14}C]glucose was detected (see Fig. 4).

Thus, amiloride is able to block sodium transport and to increase the activity of the hexosemonophosphate shunt pathway. The effect is exerted from the mucosal bathing medium from which amiloride does not enter the cells (*Robbie*, 1971). In contrast, amiloride enters and accumulates in the cells from the serosal side but has no effect upon the shunt

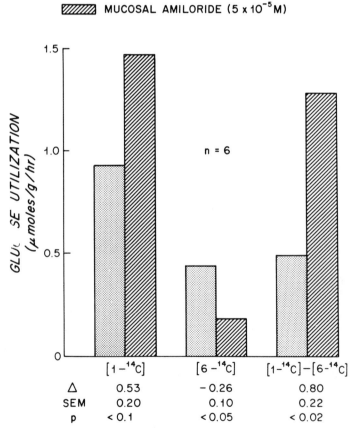

Fig. 3. Effects of amiloride, applied to the mucosal side of toad bladder, on the evolution of $^{14}CO_2$ from [1-^{14}C] and [6-^{14}C]glucose.

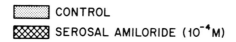

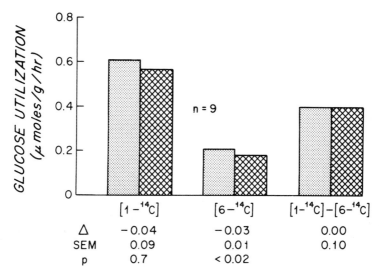

Fig. 4.   Effects of amiloride, applied to the serosal side of toad bladder, on the evolution of $^{14}CO_2$ from [1-^{14}C] and [6-^{14}C]glucose.

pathway. These effects of aldosterone and amiloride demonstrate a remarkable association between the apical cell membrane, sodium transport and the metabolism of glucose via the hexosemonophosphate shunt pathway.

REFERENCES

Baba, W., Lant, A., Smith, A., Townshend, M., and Wilson, G. 1968. Pharmacological effects in animals and normal human subjects of the diuretic amiloride-HCl. Clin Pharm Ther 9:318–327

Beckman, B., Guertler, B., Leaf, R., Witkum, P.A., and Sharp, G.W.G. 1974. Evidence for an apical membrane effect in the regulation of the hexose monophosphate shunt pathway in toad bladder. Studies with amiloride. Biochim Biophys Acta 332:350–357

Bentley, P.J. 1968. Amiloride. A potent inhibitor of sodium transport across the toad bladder. J Physiol 195:317–330

Ehrlich, E.N. and Crabbé, J. 1968. The mechanism of action of amipramizide. Pflügers Arch 302:79–96

Eigler, J., Kelter, J., and Renner, E. 1967. Effective properties of a new acyl-guanidine—amiloride-HCl(MK 870)—in the isolated skin of amphibians Klin Woch 45:737–738

Kirchberger, M.A., Chen, L.C., and Sharp, G.W.G. 1971. Further studies on the effect of aldosterone on glucose metabolism in toad bladder. Biochim Biophys Acta 241:861–875

Kirchberger, M.A., Martin, D.G., Leaf, A., and Sharp, G.W.G. 1968. The effect of aldosterone on glucose metabolism in toad bladder. Biochim Biophys Acta 165:22–31

Robbie, D.R. 1971. Studies on the mode of action of aldosterone. Ph.D. Thesis. Harvard Medical School

Sharp, G.W.G., and Leaf, A. 1964. Biological action of aldosterone *in vitro*. Nature 202:1185–1188

Sharp, G.W.G., and Leaf, A. 1965. Metabolic requirements for sodium transport stimulated by aldosterone. J Biol Chem 240:4816–4821

Wood, H.G., Katz, J., and Landau, B.R. 1963. Estimation of pathways of carbohydrate metabolism. Biochem Zeit 338:809–847

Amiloride and Epithelial Sodium Transport
Edited by A.W. Cuthbert, G.M. Fanelli, Jr. and A. Scriabine

Does Aldosterone Modify the Response of Target Tissues to Amiloride?

J. Crabbé

Departments of Physiology and Medicine
University of Louvain
(U.C.L.) Medical School
Brussels, Belgium

Eigler, Kelter, and *Renner* (1967) were first to report that amiloride blocks sodium transport by the isolated frog skin both quickly and reversibly when applied to the outer surface of the preparation. As a mechanism of action, it was proposed soon thereafter that the drug prevents sodium from interacting with specific sites at the apical pole of epithelial cells specialized in transcellular sodium transport (*Bentley,* 1968; *Ehrlich* and *Crabbé,* 1968). *Cuthbert et al.* (see Amiloride as a Membrane Probe, this volume) furthered these conclusions, providing evidence for amiloride binding to such sites (see also *Benos* and *Mandel,* 1978).

Amiloride seemingly acts mainly, if not only, on those epithelia capable of transporting sodium against highly unfavorable electrochemical potential gradients (see *Bentley,* The Comparative Pharmacology of Amiloride, this volume). In mammals, this is the case for the distal parts of the nephron, the intestinal tract and the ducts draining saliva. In amphibia, the drug has been shown to act on abdominal skin, urinary bladder and colon. By contrast, the drug fails to interfere with sodium transport in the small intestine of *Bufo marinus* (Fig. 1).

Interestingly, those amphibian epithelia sensitive to amiloride also respond to aldosterone by an increase in their sodium-transporting activity. Furthermore, the specialized channels (broadly speaking) through which sodium crosses the apical pole of the cells forming these

---

Amiloride was generously provided by Merck, Sharp and Dohme, Ltd., and aldosterone by CIBA-Geigy.

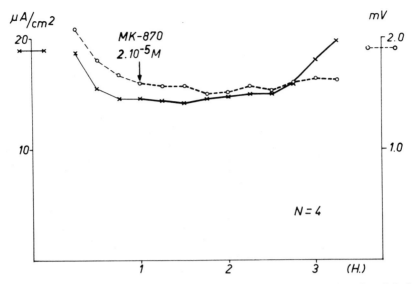

Fig. 1.   Small intestine of *Bufo marinus*. In four instances, the small intestine of *Bufo marinus* was studied *in vitro* according to *Ussing* and *Zerahn* (1951) before and after addition of amiloride (MK-870) to the luminal side of the preparation. Glucose, 10 mM, had been added to the Ringer's solution for these incubations. No change in the electrical parameters resulted from the presence of amiloride at concentrations amply sufficient to block sodium transport by more distal segments of the toad's intestinal tract (*Ehrlich* and *Crabbé*, 1968).

epithelia have been considered as one of the possible sites of action of aldosterone (for a review, see *Crabbé*, 1977). Therefore, it was thought that amiloride could help shed additional light on this issue, on the basis of the following reasoning: If the hormonal action were exerted at the basolateral membrane, no change in interaction between drug and tissue would be expected, nor would there be any change if aldosterone modified the situation at the apical site only quantitatively, e.g., by a multiplication of the sodium channels. On the other hand, if the latter were influenced *qualitatively*, a change in sensitivity to amiloride would result. A brief account of these results has appeared previously (*Crabbé*, and *Scarlata*, 1969).

Thus, the effect of amiloride was evaluated in amphibian epithelia (frog skin, toad bladder and skin) studied by the short-circuit technique (*Ussing* and *Zerahn*, 1951) after stimulation of aldosterone secretion prior to sacrifice or after incubation in the presence of the hormone.

For most experiments, the results of which will be discussed, the effect of amiloride was evaluated by interpolation, so as to take into account fluctuations in baseline activity (Fig. 2).

ALDOSTERONE *IN VIVO*

It is known that modifications in the availability of sodium in the toad's environment lead to changes in blood aldosterone concentrations, which in turn influence the rate of sodium transport by skin and bladder (*Crabbé*, 1977). Actually, when toads were maintained for a few days in dilute saline vs water, short-circuit current averaged 22.2 vs 31.7 μA/cm^2 (there were 20 animals in each group). Upon addition of amiloride, 0.4

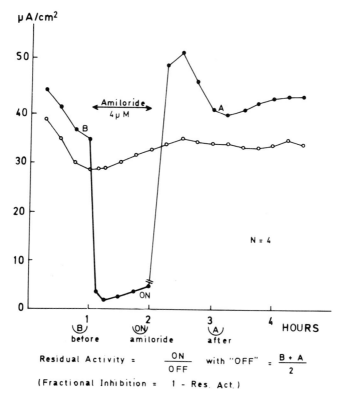

Fig. 2.   Effect of amiloride on sodium transport. Two symmetrical pieces of the abdominal skin of the toad *Bufo marinus* (originating from South America) were incubated simultaneously according to *Ussing* and *Zerahn* (1951) in Ringer's fluid (115 mM NaCl, 2.5 mM KHCO$_3$ and 1 mM CaCl$_2$) aerated with ambient air. After 1 hr, amiloride was added to the solution on the outside of one of the paired preparations. One hr later, the drug-containing solution was removed and incubation proceeded after appropriate rinsing. Final concentration of amiloride was in this instance one order of magnitude larger than that bringing about a 50% reduction approximately of sodium-transporting activity, by toad bladder (*Bentley*, 1968) or frog skin (*Cuthbert* and *Shum*, 1974). In the presence of the drug, short-circuit current across those preparations is still a reliable expression of net, active sodium transport (*Ehrlich* and *Crabbé*, 1968).

μM, residual activity averaged 0.44 $\pm$ 0.03 vs 0.60 $\pm$ 0.03, the difference being significant at P < 0.001.

Bladders behaved similarly, although the difference between mean residual activities failed to reach statistical significance, values being 0.59 $\pm$ 0.05 and 0.70 $\pm$ 0.03 (t = 1.74). Thus, preparations stimulated by withdrawal of sodium from the animal's habitat, a manipulation which results in higher plasma aldosterone concentration, appear less sensitive to amiloride. This tentative conclusion was examined more closely on tissue stimulated after incubation with aldosterone.

ALDOSTERONE *IN VITRO*

In 20 instances, toad skin was incubated overnight in the presence of aldosterone, 5 μM, a matched piece serving as reference. The following morning, short-circuit current averaged 10.3 μA/cm^2 in controls and 16.1 μA/cm^2 for hormone-treated preparations; mean residual activities upon addition of amiloride, 0.4 μM, were 0.62 and 0.77, respectively (difference: 0.15 $\pm$ 0.03; P < 0.001).

The decreased responsiveness to amiloride on the part of tissue exposed to aldosterone also could be demonstrated when preparations were exposed to aldosterone while treated with amiloride throughout, as appears from Table 1. Indeed, the hormonal effect was more marked in relative terms in the presence of amiloride than after removal of the drug.

The abdominal skin of the frog, *Rana esculenta*, also exhibited decreased sensitivity to amiloride, 0.4 μM, after incubation overnight in the presence of aldosterone, 50 nM, since residual activities averaged 0.61 for controls and 0.75 for hormone-stimulated matched preparations

Table 1.   Decreased Effect of Amiloride on Sodium Transport by Aldosterone-stimulated Toad Skin (12 experiments)

| | Short-circuit Current (μA/cm^2 $\pm$ SE) | | | | |
| | Initial | With Amiloride (4 μM) | | | Residual activity† |
		1st hr	16 hr later	Final*	
Untreated	36.5 $\pm$ 7.6	4.4 $\pm$ 0.6	3.8 $\pm$ 0.8	20.7 $\pm$ 7.4	0.299
Aldosterone	32.0 $\pm$ 7.5	4.3 $\pm$ 1.3	16.2 $\pm$ 5.0	40.8 $\pm$ 10.3	0.526
					Δ 0.227
					$\pm$ 0.056 (SE)

* 1 hr after removal of the solution containing amiloride.

† Calculated from SCC read immediately before removal of amiloride as a function of SCC 1 hr later.

From *Ehrlich* and *Crabbé*, Pflügers Arch 302:79–96, 1968.

(Δ: 0.14 ± 0.04; N = 6; P < 0.02). Baseline short-circuit current was a mean 19.5 vs 29.6 μA/cm² for aldosterone-treated tissues.

Similar observations were made in the case of toad bladder. When one out of paired hemibladders was stimulated by overnight exposure to 5 μM aldosterone, mean short-circuit current rose from 7.4 to 13.4 μA/cm². Residual activity with 0.5 μM amiloride averaged 0.68 vs 0.45 for control. The difference of 0.23 ± 0.08 is statistically significant (N = 10; P < 0.02).

On the other hand, a decreased sensitivity to amiloride could not be demonstrated in acute experiments with aldosterone (see also *Robbie*, 1971). After incubation of fresh preparations for 4 hr in the presence of the hormone, 50 nM, residual activity on 0.4 μM amiloride was 0.51 vs 0.53; admittedly, current had increased by a mere 5.0 ± 1.5 μA/cm² (N = 10) as a result of aldosterone treatment. The latter proved more effective when started after overnight incubation (at room temperature in the absence of glucose) since current doubled in 4 hr, increasing by 9.5 ± 3.4 μA/cm² (N = 8); yet residual activity on 0.4 μM amiloride averaged 0.56 and 0.66 (Δ: 0.10 ± 0.07; P < 0.2).

The reason for the discrepancy between acute and "chronic" studies is not apparent. This is the more so that bladders exposed by *Bentley* (1968) to aldosterone, 10 μM, for 4 hr after a pre-incubation at 5°C during 18 hr, proved less sensitive to amiloride, since in the presence of the drug (10 μM), short-circuit current dropped in 10 min to 36% of baseline in the case of control preparations, the corresponding value for hormone-stimulated ones being 48%.

Another, perhaps less frustrating attempt consisted of treating fresh hemibladders with aldosterone in the presence of amiloride, 1 μM. In these conditions short-circuit current increased over 3 hr from 8.6 to 20.4 μA/cm², whereas corresponding values for matched preparations were 7.6 and 16.1 μA/cm². The sodium-transporting activity of hormone-exposed preparations increased 3.3-fold, vs 2.8 for matched control (Δ: 0.46 ± 0.27; P < 0.2; N = 8).

The progressive rise in current noted for preparations exposed continuously to amiloride is a standard observation; it occurs also when sodium transport is decreased by reducing the ion's concentration in the solution on the outside, in sharp contrast to the progressive drop seen with ouabain (Fig. 3).

AMILORIDE SENSITIVITY AND THE LEVEL OF Na TRANSPORT

Is decreased sensitivity of aldosterone-stimulated amphibian epithelia to amiloride a mere consequence of increased sodium-transporting activity?

Before concluding from the preceding discussion that aldosterone

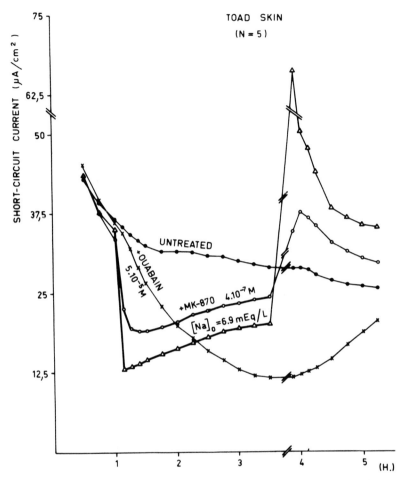

Fig. 3. The pattern for short-circuit current with amiloride (MK-870) and with low sodium Ringer compared with ouabain treatment. In five instances, four pieces of the abdominal skin of freshly killed *Bufo marinus* were incubated simultaneously in Ringer's fluid according to *Ussing* and *Zerahn* (1951). After 1 hr, amiloride (MK-870) was added to the solution on the outside in one instance; in another, sodium concentration on the outside was reduced by dilution with sodium-free Ringer's (Na Cl being replaced with Mg Cl₂); in a third instance, ouabain was added to the solution on the inside. The fourth piece served as a reference. Almost 3 hr later, incubation was resumed in the standard conditions. The pattern for current with amiloride resembled that which resulted from temporary sodium withdrawal. When a cardiac glycoside was used to interfere with sodium transport, the profile was strikingly different.

Table 2. Effect of Amiloride on Sodium Transport by Toad Bladder and Skin Stimulated by Hypotonicity

Tonicity of Incubation Fluid on Serosal Side (Osm/kg H$_2$O)	Sodium-transporting Activity by					
	Bladder (N = 6)			Skin (N = 6)		
	SCC(μA/cm^2)			SCC(μA/cm^2)		
	Off	On*	Residual Activity	Off	On†	Residual Activity
	Amiloride			Amiloride		
0.225	18.1	13.7	0.71	28.3	12.2	0.42
0.115	29.4	21.5	0.72	33.8	15.5	0.46

* 0.4 μM, for 45 min.
† 0.5 μM, for 60 min.

brings about a change in the characteristics of the sodium channels at the apical pole of target cells, it should be demonstrated that sodium-transporting activity does not regulate *per se* the responsiveness to amiloride.

After incubation overnight of those skin preparations from water- vs saline-exposed toads, whereby a steroid-depleted state could be achieved, amiloride was *more* effective on more active preparations, in terms of short-circuit current (r = 0.45; N = 34).

The electrical activity of amphibian epithelia can be stimulated by exposing their inner surface to hypotonic solution (*Ussing*, 1965). Reducing by one-half the concentration of sodium chloride in Ringer's fluid brought about an increase in short-circuit current (Table 2), more pronounced for toad bladder than skin.

As can be seen, no change in sensitivity to amiloride could be demonstrated in the above conditions.

Table 3. Sensitivity to Amiloride of Toad Skin Treated with Insulin or Aldosterone

Hormonal Treatment	Short-circuit Current (μA/cm^2)		Residual Activity
	Off	On	
	Amiloride		
None	9.8	5.3	0.53
+ Aldosterone	16.0	11.1	0.68*
+ Insulin	23.9	12.4	0.53

The abdominal skin from eight toads was divided into three pieces incubated overnight, one of them in the presence of aldosterone, 5μM. The following morning, one of the two untreated pieces was exposed to insulin, 0.125 U/ml, 1 hr prior to addition of amiloride, 0.4 μM, to all preparations for 45 min.

*Statistically different from control (Δ: 0.15 $\pm$ 0.04; P < 0.01).

Insulin is another hormone capable of bringing about a lasting stimulation of sodium transport by toad skin *in vitro* (*André* and *Crabbé*, 1966). Sensitivity to amiloride of preparations treated with insulin was not different from that of control, unlike that obtained for matched ones stimulated with aldosterone (Table 3).

Thus, the decrease in response to amiloride documented for aldosterone-stimulated amphibian epithelia seems to be induced by the hormone. *Cuthbert* and *Shum* (1975) have reported that the number of binding sites for amiloride of fresh toad bladder exposed to aldosterone 0.5 μM for 4 hr, increased. No change in amiloride affinity was found in aldosterone-treated tissues, as reported here with treatment of the same duration.

INFLUENCE OF GLUCOSE ON THE RESPONSE OF ALDOSTERONE-STIMULATED AMPHIBIAN EPITHELIA TO AMILORIDE

Energy-providing substrates enhance markedly the effect of aldosterone on sodium transport by amphibian epithelia after prolonged incubation (*Porter* and *Edelman*, 1964). It was considered of interest to evaluate this situation with respect to sensitivity to amiloride, as it is not easy to visualize how such a substrate effect could result from changes in the functional properties of the sodium channels with which the apical border of epithelia sensitive to aldosterone are equipped.

Addition of glucose, 10 mM, led an increase in the sodium-transporting activity of those toad skins dealt with above from 16.1 to 41.0 μA/cm². Residual activity with amiloride, 0.4 μM, averaged 0.77 before glucose and decreased to 0.68 thereafter (Δ: 0.09 $\pm$ 0.02; $P <$ 0.001; $N = 20$). On the other hand, when the sensitivity to amiloride was calculated from the glucose-induced *increase* in current, the value of 0.61 was arrived at, equal to that of 0.62 obtained for matched untreated preparations.

This provides an experimental argument against glucose somehow influencing the apical border of sodium-transporting cells stimulated by aldosterone.

The tentative conclusion of these observations is that aldosterone acts in such a way that the apical border of responsive epithelia grows less sensitive to amiloride, suggesting that, under hormonal influence, sodium channels exhibiting a preference for the ion vs amiloride are set into action. In other words, the question raised in the title of this paper can be answered in the affirmative.

REFERENCES

André R., and Crabbé, J.   1966.   Stimulation by insulin of active sodium transport by toad skin. Influence of aldosterone and vasopressin. Arch int Physiol Biochim 73:538–540

Benos, D.J., and Mandel, L.J.   1978.   Irreversible inhibition of sodium entry sites in frog skin by a photosensitive amiloride analog. Science 199:1205–1206

Bentley, P.J.   1968.   Amiloride. A potent inhibitor of sodium transport across the toad bladder. J Physiol (Lond) 195:317–330

Bentley, P.J.   1979.   The Comparative Pharmacology of Amiloride. In *Amiloride and Epithelial Sodium Transport*, eds. A.W. Cuthbert, G.M. Fanelli, Jr. and A. Scriabine, Baltimore: Urban & Schwarzenberg

Crabbé, J.   1977.   The Mechanism of Action of Aldosterone. In *Receptors and Mechanism of Action of Steroid Hormones*, Part II, Chap. 10, ed. J.R. Pasqualini, pp. 513–568. Modern Pharmacology-Toxicology, Vol 8, New York: Marcel Dekker, Inc.

Crabbé, J., and Scarlata, J.   1969.   Atténuation par l'aldosterone de l'effect inhibiteur exercé par l'amiloride sur le transport actif du sodium par les epitheliums d'amphibian. J de Physiol (Paris) 61:254

Cuthbert, A.W.   1979.   Amiloride as a Membrane Probe. In *Amiloride and Epithelial Sodium Transport*, eds. A.W. Cuthbert, G.M. Fanelli, Jr. and A. Scriabine, Baltimore: Urban & Schwarzenberg

Cuthbert, W.W., and Shum, W.K.   1974.   Amiloride and the sodium channel. Naunyn-Schmiedeberg's Arch Pharmacol 281:261–269

Cuthbert, A.W., and Shum, W.K.   1975.   Effects of vasopressin and aldosterone on amiloride binding in toad bladder epithelial cells. Proc R Soc B 189:543–575

Ehrlich, E.N., and Crabbé, J.   1968.   The mechanism of action of amipramizide. Pflügers Arch 302:79–96

Eigler, J., Kelter, J., and Renner, E.   1967.   Wirkungscharakteristika eines neuen Acylguanidins—Amiloride-HCl (MK 870)—an der isolierten Haut von Amphibien. Klin Wschr 45:737–738

Porter, G.A., and Edelman, I.S.   1964.   The action of aldosterone and related corticosteroids on sodium transport across the toad bladder. J Clin Invest 43:611–620

Robbie, D.R.   1971.   "Studies on the Mechanism of Action of Aldosterone: the Induction Hypothesis," Ph.D. Thesis, Cambridge, Mass (USA)

Ussing, H.H.   1965.   Relationship between osmotic reactions and active sodium transport in the frog skin epithelium. Acta Physiol Scand 63:141–155

Ussing, H.H., and Zerahn, K.   1951.   Active transport of sodium as the source of electric current in the short-circuited isolated frog skin. Acta Physiol Scand 23:110–127

An X-Ray Microanalysis of Cellular Electrolytes in Frog Skin Epithelium: The Site of Action of Amiloride and the Pathway of Na*

*A. Dörge, R. Rick, R. Bauer, Ch. Roloff, E. v.Arnim
and K. Thurau*

*Physiologisches Institut der Universität München
Pettenkoferstrasse 12
8 München 2, W. Germany*

All the models developed so far to describe the process of transepithelial Na transport are based on the assumption that Na, which is actively transported, has to pass two barriers: one at the apical and one at the basal cell membrane. Following the fundamental work of *Koefoed-Johnsen* and *Ussing* (1958) on frog skin, the entrance of Na into the cellular transport compartment across the apical membrane (outside) has been considered to be a passive step, whereas the extrusion of Na at the basolateral membranes (inside) is ascribed to an active transport process. However, in amphibian epithelia, e.g., frog skin and toad urinary bladder, which are composed of different cell layers and types, localizing the two barriers to Na movement and the Na transport compartment is far from straightforward. For this reason, attempts during the last 20 years to locate the Na transport compartment within the frog skin epithelium have given rise to conflicting results (*Cereijido* and *Rotunno*, 1968; *Koefoed-Johnsen* and *Ussing*, 1958; *Ussing* and *Windhager*, 1964; *Voûte* and *Ussing*, 1968, 1970).

However, by confining measurements of electrolyte composition to single cells of an epithelium at different states of Na transport, it should

* Supported by the Deutsche Forschungsgemeinschaft.

be possible to locate the Na transport compartment. In this connection, the diurectic substance, amiloride, could play a decisive role, since numerous experiments employing different techniques have indicated that the inhibitory effect of amiloride upon transepithelial Na transport is due only to an inhibition of the passive transport step at the outer barrier (*Bentley*, 1968; *Cuthbert*, 1973; *Dörge* and *Nagel*, 1970; *Ehrlich* and *Crabbé*, 1968; *Eigler*, *Kelter*, and *Renner*, 1967; *Moreno et al.*, 1973; *Nagel* and *Dörge*, 1970; *Rick*, *Dörge*, and *Nagel*, 1975).

The present paper is concerned with experiments in which amiloride was used in conjunction with other substances to alter the transepithelial Na transport, and then the resulting intracellular electrolyte concentrations were measured using electron microprobe analysis. Such measurements should provide further information regarding the mode and site of action of amiloride and the size and location of the Na transport compartment.

METHOD

The experiments were performed in Ussing-type chambers under short-circuited conditions on the skin of *Rana temporaria* and *R. esculenta*. At the end of the incubation period each skin was removed from the chamber, the outside surface covered with a thin layer of albumin Ringer's solution and the epithelium and adherent albumin frozen in liquid propane at $-180°C$. Cryosections of about 1 μm thickness were cut perpendicular to the surface (Reichert OMU 2) and then freeze-dried at $-80°C$. The analysis of the sections was performed in a scanning electron microscope (Cambridge S4) with an energy-dispersive X-ray detector system (EDAX; Link). Figure 1 illustrates the principle of the measuring technique. Incident electrons generate X-rays in the specimen, which are recorded by the X-ray detector as an energy spectrum in a pulse height analyzer. Simultaneously, an image is formed by the transmitted electrons so that the site of analysis can be visualized. A more detailed description of this method has been published elsewhere (*Dörge et al.*, 1978).

RESULTS AND DISCUSSION

Figure 2 shows a scanning transmission electron micrograph of a freeze-dried section of frog skin in which the different cell layers, i.e., stratum corneum, granulosum, spinosum and germinativum, are discernible. The section also contains one mitochondria-rich cell, with a characteristic pear-like shape, which interrupts the typical arrangement of the cell layers. Also shown are two spectra obtained from an extracellular and intracellular space. The upper spectrum, which has been obtained in the albumin standard layer adherent to the epithelial surface, shows the pat-

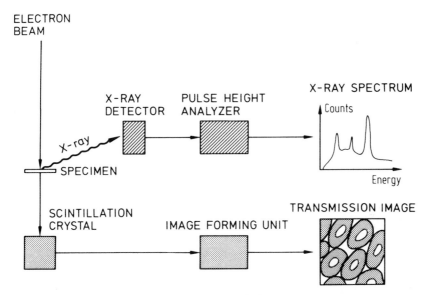

Fig. 1.   Schematic representation of X-ray microanalysis.

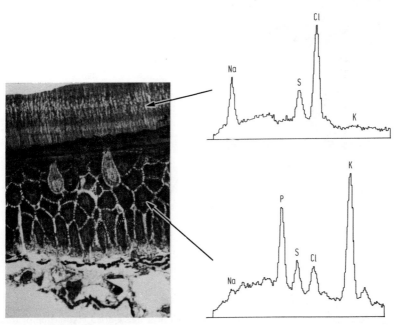

Fig. 2.   Scanning transmission electron micrograph of a freeze-dried cryosection of frog skin epithelium (about 1-μm thick) and two X-ray spectra obtained in the albumin standard layer and in a spiny cell.

tern typical for extracellular electrolytes, whereas the lower spectrum, taken from a spiny cell, exhibits a pattern typical for the intracellular composition of electrolytes. Compared to the extracellular spectrum, the intracellular spectrum shows lower Na and Cl and higher P and K peaks. Quantification was performed by comparing the elemental characteristic peaks of the specimen with those of the standard Ringer's solution. The Na peak of the albumin standard spectrum corresponds to 130, the Cl peak to 95 and the K peak to 2.5 mmole/kg wet wt.

Under control conditions, similar X-ray spectra as in the spiny cell were obtained in almost all cell types of frog skin, except in the cornified cells of the stratum corneum and in a special type of light and swollen cells occasionally appearing in the first layer beneath the stratum corneum. As can be seen from Figure 3, both the cornified cells of the stratum corneum and the light cells of the stratum granulosum showed typical extracellular electrolyte compositions. Compared to the extracellular albumin standard spectrum, the spectra of both structures show similar intensities in their Na, Cl and K peaks. The electrolyte

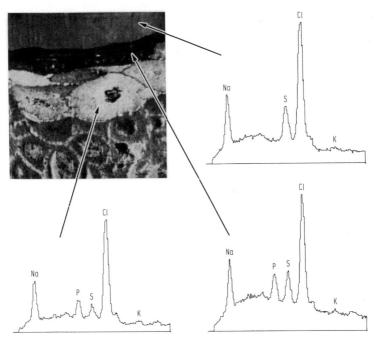

Fig. 3. Scanning transmission electron micrograph of a freeze-dried cryosection of frog skin epithelium (about 1-μm thick) and three X-ray spectra obtained in the albumin standard layer (upper spectrum), the stratum corneum (lower spectrum, right) and a light cell of the first living cell layer (lower spectrum, left).

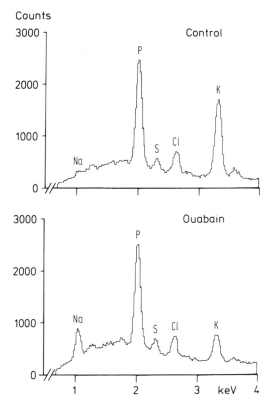

Fig. 4. Cellular X-ray spectra obtained in the stratum spinosum under control conditions and after ouabain (10^{-4}M; 90 min).

concentrations of these cellular structures were diminished to almost zero when the outside of the skin was bathed in distilled water, but were not altered after the application of substances like ouabain or amiloride. Therefore, it might be concluded that these cells represent an extracellular compartment and are not at all involved in transepithelial Na transport.

In a first set of experiments, the transepithelial Na transport was inhibited by blocking the active transport step at the inside with the use of ouabain. After the application of ouabain at a concentration of 10^{-4} M to the inside, the short-circuit current decreased within 40–60 min to between 5 and 10% of the control values. Figure 4 shows two X-ray spectra of cells in the stratum spinosum under control conditions and after incubation with ouabain. Compared to the control spectrum, the spectrum after ouabain shows an increase in Na and a decrease in K concentration. Similar increases in the Na peak and decreases in the K

106   Dörge et al.

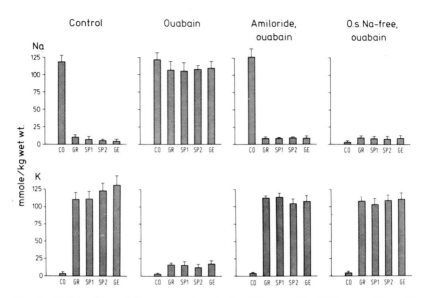

Fig. 5. Cellular Na and K concentrations in the different epithelial layers of frog skin under control conditions, after ouabain, during simultaneous application of ouabain and amiloride, and when the outside was incubated with Na-free Ringer's solution. CO = corneum; GR = granulosum; SP1 and SP2 = superficial and deeper spinosum; GE = germinativum. Values respresent mean ± 2 SEM. From *Rick et al.*, J Membrane Biol 39:313–331, 1978.

peak could be observed in all epithelial cell layers after ouabain. The average Na concentration increased after ouabain from 10 to 110 mmole/kg wet wt, and the K concentration decreased by nearly the same amount from 120 to 18 mmole/kg wet wt.

In order to clarify the origin of the accumulated cellular Na after ouabain, the action of ouabain was studied in the presence of amiloride. Amiloride was applied at a concentration of 10^{-4} M to the outside. Figure 5 shows the Na and K concentrations of the different cell layers under control conditions, after ouabain and during application of amiloride simultaneous to ouabain. As already described, after the action of ouabain the Na concentration increased in all epithelial cell layers except the stratum corneum by about 100 mmole/kg wet wt, whereas the K concentration decreased to almost the same extent. However, when amiloride was applied in addition to ouabain, the Na concentration remained low and the K concentration high, as under control conditions. Similar results were obtained when during the application of ouabain, the outside was bathed with Na-free Ringer's solution. The results demonstrate that the cellular accumulation of Na after ouabain is caused by an influx of Na from the outside bathing solution. Since amiloride or Na-free solutions at the outside inhibit the increase in Na concentration after ouabain in all epithelial cell layers, it must be concluded that the site of action of amiloride is situated at the outer membrane of the outermost living cell layer.

Figure 6 illustrates an experiment demonstrating that the effect of ouabain can even be reversed when after 60 min of its application, the outside Ringer's solution is replaced by Na-free solution; moreover, this reversal can be almost abolished by the action of amiloride. After ouabain the typical increase in the Na concentration and the simultaneous decrease in the K concentration can be observed in all cell layers. When the outside bathing medium was replaced with Na-free solution, both the cellular Na and K concentrations returned to control values. However, when the Na-free solution at the outside also contained amiloride this effect was hardly apparent, for the Na and K concentrations were only slightly altered compared to those occurring after ouabain alone. Therefore, it must be concluded that the reversal effect cannot be explained by a residual transport activity which extrudes Na toward the inside but is due to a passive efflux of Na to the outside, which can be blocked by amiloride.

According to the present results, all the cells of the various epithelial layers excepting the stratum corneum show the characteristic features of a Na transport compartment. Since, for the frog skin epithelium, the

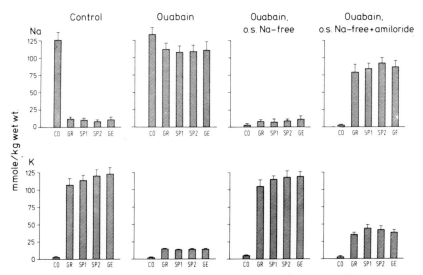

Fig. 6. Cellular Na and K concentrations in the different epithelial layers of frog skin under control conditions, after ouabain, when after 90-min incubation with ouabain the outer bathing medium was replaced with Na-free Ringer's solution, and when this solution also contained amiloride. For abbreviations of strata, see Figure 5. Values represent mean ± 2 SEM. From *Rick et al.*, J Membrane Biol 39:313–331, 1978.

extracellular pathway is sealed by the tight junctions connecting the cells of the outermost living layer (*Erlij,* 1971; *Farquhar* and *Palade,* 1965), the finding that all cell layers exchange Na mainly with the outside bathing medium supports the existence of a syncitial transport compartment, as suggested by *Ussing* and *Windhager* (1964).

To further characterize the Na transport compartment of the frog skin, the action of vasopressin upon the electrolyte concentrations of the epithelial cells was examined. Vasopressin is thought to enhance net Na transport by increasing the Na permeability of the outer-facing membranes (*Biber* and *Cruz,* 1973; *Cereijido* and *Rotunno,* 1971, *Civan* and *Frazier,* 1968; *Finn,* 1968). The arginine vasopressin concentration used was 0.2 U/ml. The increase in short-circuit current which occurred during the action of arginine vasopressin was found to vary considerably from one skin to another.

Figure 7 shows the Na and K concentrations obtained in the different cell layers of a skin in which the short-circuit current was increased by 150% after the application of arginine vasopressin to the inner side. Compared to the control, after vasopressin the Na concentrations increased in all epithelial cell layers from about 10 to 30 mmole/kg wet wt, whereas the K concentrations decreased by almost the same

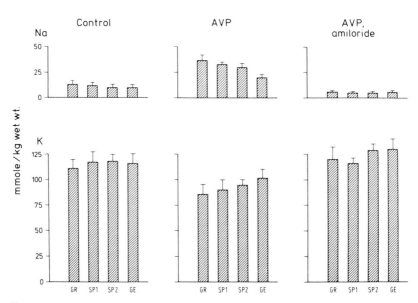

Fig. 7. Cellular Na and K concentrations in the different epithelial layers of frog skin under control conditions, after arginine vasopressin, and when after 90-min incubation with arginine vasopressin amiloride was applied. For abbreviations of strata, see Figure 5. Mean ± 2 SEM.

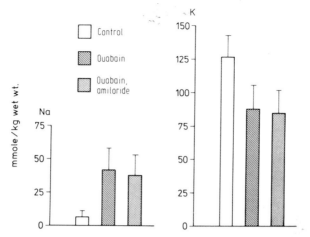

Fig. 8   Na and K concentrations of the mitochondria-rich cells under control conditions, after ouabain, and when amiloride was applied simultaneously to ouabain. Mean ± 2 SEM. From *Rick et al.*, J Membrane Biol 39:313–331,1978.

amount in all layers from about 115 to 90 mmole/kg wet wt. However, the application of amiloride at a time when the effect of arginine vasopressin upon the short-circuit current is maximal causes the short-circuit current to be reduced to almost zero and the arginine vasopressin effect upon the intracellular Na and K concentrations to be abolished. The Na concentrations decreased in all epithelial cell layers to values which are half those obtained under control conditions, whereas the K concentration increased to levels a little above those of the control. The finding that the increased Na concentration observed after the action of arginine vasopressin can be reduced in all cell layers with amiloride once again supports the view that amiloride acts at the outer-facing membrane of the outermost living cell layer and that the epithelium reacts like a syncitial Na transport compartment.

However, the conclusion that the frog skin epithelium behaves like a syncitial Na transport compartment is valid only for the cells of the different epithelial layers and does not include epithelial structures like mitochondria-rich cells and the glandular epithelium. The most striking difference between the gland and other epithelial cells was that their cellular electrolyte concentrations were almost unaffected by ouabain. The mitochondria-rich cells showed an increase in Na and a decrease in K concentrations after ouabain, which, in contrast to the other cells, was less pronounced and could not be inhibited by amiloride, as can be seen from Figure 8. The Na concentration increased on an average from 6.5 to 42, while the K concentration decreased from 127 to 88 mmole/kg wet wt. When amiloride was applied together with ouabain, the Na and K concentrations were found to be 38 and 85 mmole/kg wet wt, respectively. The effect of ouabain upon the intracellular Na concentration of the mitochondria-rich cells was found to be much less pronounced when the outer bathing medium was Na-free, indicating that part of the increase in Na concentration after ouabain in these cells is due to a Na influx from the outer side. Since amiloride does not affect the ouabain response of these cells, it appears that this Na influx is amiloride-insensitive. Thus, it can be concluded that for the frog skin, where the net transepithelial Na transport (*Dörge* and *Nagel*, 1970; *Eigler*, *Kelter*, and *Renner*, 1967) and the unidirectional Na uptake from the outside (*Moreno et al.*, 1973; *Rick*, *Dörge*, and *Nagel*, 1975) are both extremely sensitive to amiloride, the contribution of the mitochondria-rich cells to transepithelial Na transport must be negligibly small.

Figure 9 shows schematically the mode of transepithelial Na transport in frog skin as derived from the present results. Na enters the cellular compartment across the outer cell membrane of the outermost living cell layer by a passive step, which can be blocked by amiloride. Compared to the inner-facing cell membranes, this membrane is highly permeable to Na. Na passes via intercellular connections from the outer to the deeper cell layers and is extruded actively across the inner-facing cell membranes into the intercellular spaces, from which it diffuses toward the corium. However, the question as to whether all cells of the different layers are involved to the same extent in the transepithelial Na transport cannot be answered by the present experiments. It is possible that the larger part of the transepithelial Na transport is performed by a

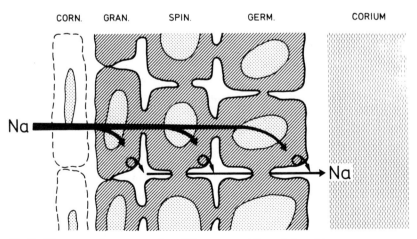

CORN.   GRAN.   SPIN.   GERM.   CORIUM

Na

Na

Fig. 9   Diagrammatic representation of Na movement through frog skin.

single cell type, to which the other cells of the epithelium are coupled (*Morel* and *Leblanc*, 1975). However, since recent studies on the distribution of ouabain binding sites (*Mills*, *Ernst*, and *DiBona*, 1977) have demonstrated that all the inner-facing membranes of the epithelium are potential sites of active Na transport, it seems more probable that each cell layer contributes significantly to transepithelial Na transport.

REFERENCES

Bentley, P.J. 1968. Amiloride: A potent inhibitor of sodium transport across the toad bladder. J Physiol (Lond) 195:317–330

Biber, T.U.L., and Cruz, L.J. 1973. Effect of antidiuretic hormone on sodium uptake across the outer surface of frog skin. Am J Physiol 225:912–917

Cereijido, M., and Rotunno, C.A. 1968. Fluxes and distribution of sodium in frog skin. A new model. J Gen Physiol 51:280–289

Cereijido, M., and Rotunno, C.A. 1971. The effect of antidiuretic hormone on Na movement across frog skin. J Physiol (Lond) 213:119–133

Civan, M.M., and Frazier, H.S. 1968. The site of the stimulatory action of vasopressin on sodium transport in toad bladder. J Gen Physiol 51:589–605

Cuthbert, A.W. 1973. An upper limit to the number of sodium channels in frog skin epithelium. J Physiol (Lond) 288:681–692

Dörge, A., and Nagel, W. 1970. Effect of amiloride on sodium transport in the frog skin. II. Sodium transport pool and unidirectional fluxes. Pflügers Arch 321:91–101

Dörge, A., Rick, R., Gehring, K., and Thurau, K. 1978. Preparation of freeze-dried cryosections for quantitative X-ray microanalysis of electrolytes in biological soft tissues. Pflügers Arch 373:85–97

Ehrlich, E.N., and Crabbé, J. 1968. The mechanism of action of amipramizide. Pflügers Arch 302:79–96

Eigler, J., Kelter, J., and Renner, E. 1967. Wirkungscharakteristika eines neuen Acylguanidins—Amiloride-HCl (MK 870)—an der isolierten Haut von Amphibien. Klin Wschr 45:737–738

Erlij, D. 1971. Salt transport across isolated frog skin. Phil Trans Roy Soc London B 262:153–161

Farquhar, M.G., and Palade, G.E. 1965. Cell junctions in amphibian skin. J Cell Biol 26:263–291

Finn, A.L. 1968. Separate effects of sodium and vasopressin on the sodium pump in toad bladder. Am J Physiol 215:849–856

Koefoed-Johnsen, V., and Ussing, H.H. 1958. The nature of the frog skin potential. Acta Physiol Scand 42:298–308

Mills, J.W., Ernst, S.A., and DiBona, D.R. 1977. Localization of Na$^+$-pump sites in frog skin. J Cell Biol 73:88–110

Morel, F., and Leblanc, G. 1975. Transient current changes and Na compartmentalization in frog skin epithelium. Pflügers Arch 358:135–157

Moreno, J.H., Reisin, I.L., Rodriguez-Boulan, E., Rotunno, C.A., and Cereijido, M. 1973. Barriers to sodium movement across frog skin. J Membrane Biol 11:99–115

Nagel, W., and Dörge, A. 1970. Effect of amiloride on sodium transport of frog skin. I. Action on intracellular sodium content. Pflügers Arch 317:84–92

Rick, R., Dörge, A., and Nagel, W.   1975.   Influx and efflux of sodium at the outer surface of frog skin. J Membrane Biol 22:183–196

Rick, R., Dörge, A., v.Arnim, E., and Thurau, K.   1978.   Electron microprobe analysis of frog skin epithelium. Evidence for a syncytial Na transport compartment. J Membrane Biol 39:313–331

Ussing, H.H., and Windhager, E.   1964.   Nature of shunt path and active sodium transport path through frog skin epithelium. Acta physiol Scand 61:484–504

Voûte, C.L., and Ussing, H.H.   1968.   Some morphological aspects of active sodium transport. The epithelium of the frog skin. J Cell Biol 36:625–638

Voûte, C.L., and Ussing, H.H.   1970.   Quantitative relation between hydrostatic pressure gradient, extracellular volume and active sodium transport in the epithelium of the frog skin (R. temporaria). Exp Cell Res 62:375–383

©1979 Urban & Schwarzenberg, Inc.   Baltimore-Munich
Amiloride and Epithelial Sodium Transport
Edited by A.W. Cuthbert, G.M. Fanelli, Jr. and A. Scriabine

Amiloride as a Membrane Probe

A. W. Cuthbert, J. M. Edwardson,
J. Aceves and S. A. Wilson

Department of Pharmacology
University of Cambridge
Hills Road, Cambridge, England

Molecules which are used as membrane probes must be able to act as reporters of the membrane structures with which they interact. The probe molecule may report directly about its environment, provided it generates a signal which is modified by interaction with its binding site. Alternatively, the probe may report directly about the number of binding sites if the material is tagged with a radioactive atom. A third way in which the probe may report is indirectly, by means of some effect it produces on the system.

Using amiloride, both direct and indirect reporting methods have been employed to investigate the sodium entry mechanisms in epithelia. However, some obvious approaches, such as using the fluorescence of the compound, are yet to be explored.

In this paper three different approaches are described in which amiloride (or an analogue) has been used to investigate the sodium entry mechanism in amphibian epithelia. In the first, the apparent affinity of amiloride as an inhibitor of sodium transport is used as an indirect indicator of the state of entry mechanism. In the second, experiments are described in which ^{14}C-amiloride binding to isolated epithelial cells from the toad bladder is used to investigate the way in which aldosterone may affect sodium transport. Finally, attempts to find a ligand superior to amiloride for use in binding studies are described, together with some preliminary results with a new compound, benzamil.

The affinity, or more correctly the apparent affinity, of a drug producing a pharmacological effect can be defined as the reciprocal of the concentration producing 50% of the maximal effect. The effects of amiloride on amphibian epithelia *in vitro* can be conveniently measured as an inhibition of the short-circuit current. Using isolated frog skin or toad urinary bladder, the curve relating inhibition of SCC to amiloride concentration approximates to a rectangular hyperbola (*Cuthbert*, 1973;

Cuthbert and *Fanelli*, 1978), and provided there is a single receptor population, the affinity will correspond to the reciprocal of the IC_{50}. In some tissues, e.g., toad colon (*Cuthbert*, 1973), and exceptionally in frog skin (*Cuthbert* and *Shum*, 1974), the concentration response curves deviate from a hyperbolic form. The deviation from a simple mass action form may indicate heterogeneity of the binding sites for amiloride, or may be indicative of cooperative effects. *Cuthbert* and *Fanelli* (1978) reported instances of tissues which gave a hyperbolic relationship for amiloride, but a more complex relationship for the analogue without the 6-chloro substituent.

Manipulations which modify the level of sodium transport and at the same time affect the apparent affinity of amiloride are of particular interest since they indicate some alteration in the properties of the entry mechanism at the apical surface of the epithelium.

It is already known that when the sodium concentration is lowered in the apical bathing solution, the apparent affinity for amiloride is increased. The relationship between the sodium concentration and affinity of amiloride is such as to suggest that the ion and amiloride interact competitively (*Cuthbert* and *Shum*, 1974). What is more interesting is that a number of other substances which affect sodium transport, but not by a direct action on the apical surface, can also affect the affinity of amiloride. For example, antidiuretic hormone, acting on receptors at the serosal surface, brings about changes resulting in an increase of sodium transport associated with a permeability increase at the apical surface. The affinity of amiloride is reduced in tissues in which sodium transport is increased by this hormone (*Cuthbert* and *Shum*, 1974). There is much biophysical evidence to indicate that the final effector site which is influenced by the hormone is the apical surface (see *De Sousa*, 1975 for references) and it is likely that the change in amiloride affinity is probing the same final effector process. Failure to detect an increase in the number of entry sites at the time transport is increased by ADH gave rise to the suggestion that the hormone increases the fraction of sites which are conducting at any instant, resulting in a reduction in the macroscopic affinity of amiloride (*Cuthbert*, 1974).

Two further examples of affinity change are given here. Sodium transport in frog skin can be stimulated by isoprenaline added to serosal fluid, (*Jard*, 1974) and acting on receptors on the serosal surface of the epithelium. Yet at the time transport is increased, the apparent affinity is reduced, indicating that whatever mechanism is activated by isoprenaline, the final effector process probably involves the apical surface of the cells. The changes in both transport and affinity of amiloride are reversible when isoprenaline is removed (Fig. 1). Theophylline also increases

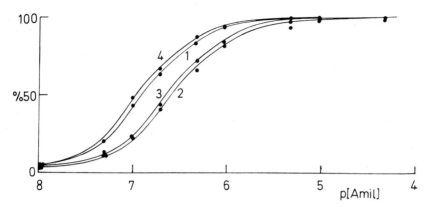

Fig. 1. Relation between percentage inhibition of short-circuit current and concentration of amiloride. The curves were determined in the order 1, 2, 3 and 4. Initial values of SCC were 102, 186, 186 and 90 μA, respectively, in 1 to 4. In 2 and 3 SCC was stimulated by the addition of isoprenaline, 100 nM, added to the serosal fluid. Skin area 3 cm², *Rana temporaria*. (Unpublished experiment by S.A. Wilson.)

sodium transport and reduces the affinity of amiloride, as shown in Figure 2.

One obvious question is whether the affinity of amiloride is simply a function of the level of sodium transport. ADH, isoprenaline and theophylline all increase transport and reduce affinity, while when the sodium concentration is reduced the short-circuit current falls and the affinity increases. In a study with 36 different skins, which were bathed on both sides in normal Ringer solution, there was no correlation

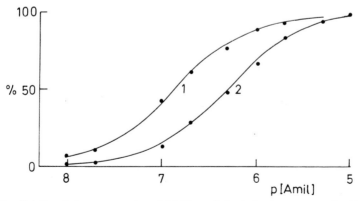

Fig. 2. Relation between percentage inhibition of short-circuit current and amiloride concentration. Initial SCC was 95 μA(curve 1), which increased to 150 μA by the addition of theophylline, 3×10^{-2} M, to both the mucosal and serosal solutions. Skin area 7 cm², *Rana temporaria*.

between basal SCC and the affinity of amiloride (*Cuthbert* and *Fanelli*, 1978).

Thus, it might be concluded that a change in amiloride affinity at a given sodium concentration may be indicative of a change in conformation or biophysical properties of the entry mechanism. Such measurements are useful at an elementary level to indicate that a change has occurred, but the nature of these changes will require a much more sophisticated approach, and it is unlikely they will be unravelled in the intact epithelium.

The effect of ADH on sodium transport in amphibian epithelia has already been alluded to. Sodium transport can also be increased in amphibian skins and bladders by aldosterone. The characteristics of the response are rather different from those with ADH. The response with aldosterone is slow to appear and takes several hours to reach a maximal value. Inhibitors of translation and transcription prevent the physiological effect of the steroid, and like other steroids, aldosterone has a nuclear site of action. *Rossier*, *Wilce*, and *Edelman* (1974) have demonstrated the formation of a class of m-RNAs in toad bladder in response to aldosterone. The important question then is how the newly synthesised protein(s) produced by translation of the aldosterone-induced message(s) affects sodium transport. The actions of aldosterone have been reviewed recently by *Crabbé* (1977) and the three major possibilities for the mechanism of action of aldosterone are the permease, pump or metabolic hypotheses. The first considers that the aldosterone-induced protein(s) (AIP) may be incorporated into the membrane as new sodium entry sites. Alternatively, the proteins may be new pumps to be incorporated into the serosal membrane. Thirdly, the AIP may represent an increased ability to produce energy available for transport. There is rather little evidence for the second hypothesis; furthermore, there appears to be a considerable excess of pump sites to deal with sodium influx. The specific activity of citrate synthase has been shown to increase following aldosterone, in line with the second hypothesis (*Law & Edelman*, 1978). There is considerable biophysical evidence to indicate the apical permeability to sodium is increased by aldosterone. Indeed, the three mechanisms are not mutually exclusive, and other as yet undiscovered mechanisms may be operative also.

The permease hypothesis has been examined using ^{14}C-amiloride as a way of determining the density of sodium entry sites in the cells of isolated toad bladder (*Cuthbert* and *Shum*, 1975). When the apical surfaces of bladders are bathed in low sodium-Ringer (1.1 mM Na), amiloride has an affinity of around 10 nM^{-1}. Addition of aldosterone increases the current by 70% or so during a 4-hr exposure without changing the affinity for amiloride.

Using suspensions of isolated toad-bladder epithelial cells in isotonic choline chloride Ringer containing 1.1 mM sodium, we were able to detect a component of binding using ^{14}C-amiloride which had the properties expected of the entry sites. Binding to this component showed saturation and had a Km equal to that when amiloride was used to inhibit transport. Furthermore, triamterene was able to displace ^{14}C-amiloride binding, again at the concentration expected from its activity on sodium transport.

The maximal number of binding sites in freshly isolated cells was 1400/μm^2. (The calculation assumes all the entry sites are concentrated onto one-sixth of the cell surface, the area exposed to the apical solution; thus, if the sites were evenly distributed, the density would be 230/μm^2.) One as yet unexplained feature of these studies was that over 4–5 hr the binding site density fell to 200–400/μm^2 and then remained constant for up to a week.

There is no conclusive way to know if the binding sites measured in this way are identical with sodium entry sites, but it can be stated that their properties are consistent with those expected from inhibition studies in intact epithelia.

To examine the effects of aldosterone bladders, halves were incubated with either aldosterone or solvent (as control), after which the cells from each bladder half were isolated and the density of displaceable amiloride binding sites measured at a single concentration.

The results for 13 separate experiments in which bladders were exposed to 5×10^{-7} M aldosterone for 4 hr are given in Table 1. The data show the number of binding sites measured using different concentrations of ^{14}C-amiloride which were displaced by a 100-fold excess of unlabeled drug. Of course, each of these experiments represents only one point on a total binding curve. Reference to the total binding curve suggests that approximately 7, 15 and 30% of the displaceable binding at the three concentrations of ^{14}C-amiloride (21.9, 43.8 and 83.8 nM) were due to nonspecific binding.

In each experiment there was an increase in the density of binding sites following aldosterone. Also, it will be noted that in the experiments using 83.8 nM ^{14}C-amiloride the initial values were lower than expected. In these experiments the toads were immersed in normal saline for 15 hr before the bladders were excised. This procedure is known to depress the levels of endogenous aldosterone, which further supports the suggestion that binding is to sodium entry sites.

Similar results are obtained at lower aldosterone concentrations (5×10^{-8} M) and when the cells are separated prior to exposure to aldosterone (Table 2).

Another way of testing if the increase in binding sites following

Table 1. Effects of Aldosterone (5 × 10^{-7} M) on ^{14}C-amiloride Binding in Isolated Epithelial Cells from Toad Bladder

Amiloride Concentration (nM)	Binding Sites per Cell (×10^5)	
	Solvent Control	Aldosterone
21.9	0.58	1.14
	0.29	0.66
	0.19	0.46
43.8	1.16	1.91
	1.53	2.24
	0.88	2.91
	0.94	1.27
	0.75	1.07
83.8	0.51	1.73
+ saline pretreatment	0.77	2.10
	0.66	1.81
	1.38	2.20
	0.58	1.08

In each experiment the bilobed bladder was separated into two lobes. One half was exposed to aldosterone and the other served as control. Cells were harvested from each lobe and labeled with amiloride 4 hr after exposure to hormone. Binding sites are calculated from the amount of binding displaced by a 100-fold excess of unlabeled amiloride. From *Cuthbert* and *Shum*, (1975).

Table 2. Effects of Aldosterone (5 × 10^{-8} M) on ^{14}C-amiloride Binding

Experiment	Binding Sites per Cell × 10^5	
	Solvent Control	Aldosterone
1	0.49	0.84
2	0.56	0.85
3	0.56	0.74
4	0.67	0.98
5	0.93	1.39

In all experiments the ^{14}C-amiloride concentration was 50 nM. In experiments 1–3 cells were isolated after the tissue was exposed to aldosterone or solvent only; in 4 and 5 isolated cell suspensions were prepared from whole bladders. These were then divided into two and one-half exposed to aldosterone and the other to solvent only. Binding sites are calculated from the amount of displacement caused by 100-fold excess of unlabeled amiloride. From *Cuthbert* and *Shum* (1976).

aldosterone is related to its effects on transport is to use inhibitors of transcription and translation. When cycloheximide and actinomycin D were used at concentrations known to block the actions of aldosterone on sodium transport, the increase in the density of amiloride binding sites was also prevented (Table 3).

Thus, in a number of ways the results with ^{14}C-amiloride binding to toad-bladder cells are consistent with the so-called permease hypothesis of aldosterone action. The results do not, of course, prove the hypothesis; neither do the results distinguish between whether AIP represents new sites to be incorporated in the membrane or whether AIP uncovers pre-existing but quiescent sites.

The density of sodium entry sites in the apical surfaces of *intact* transporting epithelia is of considerable interest. The regulation of the density and modulation of the properties of the entry sites by various perturbations may help to explain ways in which epithelia are able to regulate transport in physiological conditions. In addition, the mean turnover number and mean conductance of the entry sites can be calculated if both channel density and other biophysical parameters are known.

Table 3.   Effects of Actinomycin D (5 μg/ml) and Cycloheximide (0.5 μg/ml) on the Stimulation of ^{14}C-amiloride Binding by Aldosterone (5 $\times$ 10^{-7}M)

Experiment	Binding Sites per Cell $\times 10^5$	
	Aldosterone plus Actinomycin	Aldosterone Alone
1	0.99	1.36
2	0.89	1.43
3	0.77	1.07
4	1.16	1.71
5	0.88	1.20
	Aldosterone plus Cycloheximide	Aldosterone Alone
1	1.24	2.58
2	0.92	2.32
3	1.12	1.62
4	0.78	1.02
5	1.10	1.54

The ^{14}C-amiloride concentration was 84 nM throughout. Binding sites were calculated from the amount of displaceable binding by a 100-fold excess of unlabeled amiloride. The procedure was as for Table 1. From *Cuthbert* and *Shum* (1975).

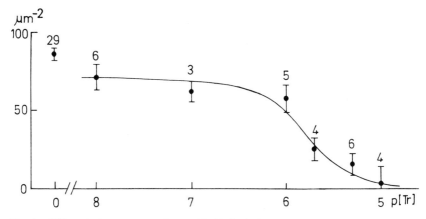

Fig. 3.   Effect of triamterene on the specific binding of ^{14}C-amiloride to frog skin. In each of 29 skins the amount of binding of ^{14}C-amiloride (10 nM) which could be displaced by a 100-fold excess of unlabeled amiloride was measured in the absence and presence of one concentration of triamterene. Redrawn from *Cuthbert* and *Shum*, Molec Pharmacol 10:880–891, 1974.

In the last four years a number of studies have been made in which the density of amiloride binding sites has been measured in isolated frog skin. The density of specifically bound amiloride (i.e., displaced by 100-fold excess of unlabeled amiloride) was taken as equivalent to the density of sodium entry sites. In these studies large areas (10 cm²) of frog skin were used, and the apical surface always was bathed in low sodium solutions to increase the affinity of amiloride (to about 10^8 M^{-1}).

The first attempt to measure a binding curve with amiloride was by *Cuthbert* and *Shum* (1974). The binding curve appeared to saturate at a site density of 90/μm² at zero sodium, but we were not satisfied that saturation was complete. Unfortunately, technical reasons prevented measurements at higher ligand concentrations. An alternative approach was to measure the specific binding at one concentration and to multiply this by the reciprocal of the fractional occupancy. The latter was estimated from the simultaneous measurement of SCC inhibition by the ligand with the apical surface bathed in low (1.1 mEq/1) sodium Ringer. The same paper reported values of around 200/μm² when measured by this method.

Part of the evidence that we were measuring binding to sodium entry sites came from using another ligand to displace amiloride, namely triamterene. Figure 3 shows the effect of triamterene on the specific (displaceable) binding of amiloride in 29 tissues. The affinity of triamterene deduced from these experiments was close to the value obtained when triamterene was used to inhibit transport (*Cuthbert* and *Shum*, 1974). The figure is reproduced here for another reason, to illustrate one of the difficulties of working with amiloride as a radiolabel. The methods used previously are extremely tedious and time consuming, and the result illustrated took 29 days of experimentation to complete, since a single control and test point in one tissue took 8 hr.

Clearly a better radioligand, with higher affinity and greater specific activity, is needed. In addition, such an improved ligand might be useful in attempts to actually isolate the channel biochemically. We started to search for such a material and present here some preliminary results with one compound.

Our search gave N-benzylamidino-3-5-diamino-6-chloropyrazine carboxamide, a benzyl derivative of amiloride which we have called benzamil. The material was labeled with tritium on the metaposition of the phenyl ring, and initially had a specific activity of 21,000 c mole^{-1}.

We have studied the binding of this material to isolated frog-skin epithelium, prepared using treatment with collagenase and mild hydrostatic pressure. Pieces (0.95 cm²) were clamped in small perspex chambers with the serosal surface downward and bathed in Ringer, pH 7.6. The upper apical surface was bathed in low sodium Ringer (1.1 mEq/l) at pH 6.5.

Figure 4 illustrates a typical experiment made using pieces of epithelium from two frogs. The apical bathing solution was low sodium (1.1 mEq/l) Ringer, pH 6.5, containing various concentrations of tritiated benzamil with or without excess amiloride, 1μM. The epithelia were

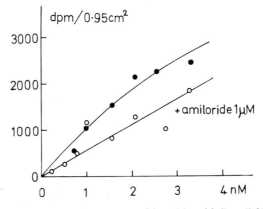

Fig. 4.   Binding of ³H-benzamil to 14 pieces of frog-skin epithelium (0.95 cm²) taken from two frogs. Closed circles are for tissues bathed in the radioligand alone, while open circles represent tissues bathed in radiolabel plus amiloride 1 μM. Lines are drawn by eye. Assuming a Km of 1.5 nM (a value obtained from inhibition of SCC by benzamil in another skin), the specific binding site density is 180/μm².

incubated with these solutions for 30–40 min, which is sufficient time for equilibrium to be established with even the lowest concentrations, after which epithelia were punched out, blotted, dissolved in Soluene 350 and counted by liquid scintillation spectrometry.

The data show some scatter which there is evidence to show is due to inequalities in the epithelial pieces themselves, but they also show clearly that there is a fraction of the total uptake which is displaceable, and that the form of the total uptake curve appears to combine a saturable and linear component. Similar pairs of curves also are obtained if the uptake of tritiated benzamil is measured at high and low sodium concentrations as indicated by Figure 5. The data for each of the last two figures could be obtained in a few hours and therefore represent a considerable methodological improvement over preceding methods with amiloride.

By considering a large number of experiments similar to the two shown above, we have used a fitting procedure to analyze the total uptake curve for tritiated benzamil at concentrations from 0 to 11 nM. The estimated value of the saturable component was 21.5 fmole cm^{-2}, corresponding to a binding site density of 130 μm^{-2} and with a half-saturating concentration of 1 nM, a value close to that estimated from inhibition of SCC by benzamil. The linear nonsaturating component had an estimated value of 10.2 fmole nM^{-1}, close to and not significantly different from the linear uptake seen in the presence of amiloride (1 μM), benzamil (1 μM) or high sodium (111 mEq/1). At pH 3.5 a linear uptake with a slope of 3.3 fmole nM^{-1} was found. At this pH approximately

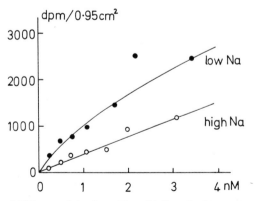

Fig. 5. Uptake of ^{3}H-benzamil by frog skin epithelium in the presence of 111 mM Na (open circles) and 1.1 mM Na (closed circles). The closed circles are mean values for two pieces; whereas, the open circles are values for a single piece of epithelium. The lines were drawn by eye. Assuming a Km value of 1.5 nM, the saturable component is equivalent to 210/μm^2.

only 3% of the sites are unprotonated (*Cuthbert*, 1976) so no saturating component is seen, but also some nonspecific binding sites are occluded.

Although the conditions used in these experiments (low sodium, pH 6.5 and open-circuit) are very different from those used previously for measuring amiloride binding, the binding site density is rather similar.

We are encouraged by these preliminary findings to feel that this new ligand may be more useful than amiloride as a membrane probe, and consider it might prove useful in the isolation of the entry mechanism.

REFERENCES

Crabbé, J. 1977. The mechanism of action of aldosterone. In *Receptors and mechanisms of action of steroid hormones*, Part II, Ed., J.R. Pasqualini, New York: Marcel Dekker, Inc

Cuthbert, A.W. 1973. Evidence for multiple forms of receptors for amiloride in transporting epithelia. Eur J Pharmacol 23:187–190

Cuthbert, A.W. 1974. Interactions of sodium channels in transporting epithelia, a two-state model. Molec Pharmacol 10:892–903

Cuthbert, A.W. 1976. Importance of guanidinium groups for blocking sodium channels in epithelia. Molec Pharmacol 12:945–957

Cuthbert, A.W. and Fanelli, G.M. 1978. Effects of some pyrazine carboxamides in sodium transport in frog skin. Brit J Pharmacol 63:139–149

Cuthbert, A.W. and Shum, W.K. 1974. Binding of amiloride to sodium channels in frog skin. Molec Pharmacol 10:880–891

Cuthbert, A.W. and Shum, W.K. 1975. Effects of vasopressin and aldosterone on amiloride binding in toad bladder epithelial cells. Proc R Soc Lond B, 189:543–575

Cuthbert, A.W. and Shum, W.K. 1976. Estimation of the lifespan of amiloride binding sites in the membranes of toad bladder epithelial cells. J Physiol 225, 605–618

De Sousa, R.C. 1975. Mécanismes de transport de l'eau et du Sodium par les cellules des epithelia d'amphibiens et du tubule rénal isolé. J Physiol (Paris), 71:5A–71A

Jard, S. 1974. Adrenergic receptors in epithelia. In *Drugs & Transport Processes*, ed. B.A. Callingham p. 111–127. London: Macmillan

Law, P.Y. and Edelman, I.S. 1978. Induction of citrate synthase by aldosterone in rat kidney. J Memb Biol *41*, 41–64

Rossier, B.C., Wilce, P.A. and Edelman, I.S. 1974. Kinetics of RNA labelling in toad bladder epithelium. Effects of aldosterone and related steroids. Proc natn Acad Sci USA, 71:3101–3105

©1979 Urban & Schwarzenberg, Inc. Baltimore-Munich
Amiloride and Epithelial Sodium Transport
Edited by A.W. Cuthbert, G.M. Fanelli, Jr. and A. Scriabine

Fluctuations Arising from Sodium Transport of Frog Skin

B. Lindemann* and W. Van Driessche**

* 2nd Department of Physiology
Universität des Saarlandes 6650
Homburg/Saar, W. Germany
** Laboratorium voor Fysiology
Universiteit te Leuven
Belgium

Epithelia are shunted two-membrane transport systems. In principle, therefore, their apical membranes, basolateral membranes and para-cellular shunts can be sources of voltage or current fluctuations. The following discussion of epithelial transport "noise" focuses on Na transport in frog skin epithelium and is based on the well-known two-membrane model, extended by inclusion of a paracellular shunt pathway (*Koefoed-Johnsen* and *Ussing*, 1958; *Ussing* and *Windhager*, 1964; *Leaf*, 1965). While the applicability of the Koefoed-Johnsen-Ussing model to amphibian epithelia recently has been challenged (*Nagel*, 1977), it also has gained defenders (*Higgins, Gebler*, and *Frömter*, 1977). Noise data have to be viewed together with macroscopic relaxation data, which are therefore included in this discussion.

OVERALL TRANSPORT PROPERTIES

Na ions are taken up passively by electrodiffusion through Na-selective channels in the apical membrane of cells (outer stratum granulosum) right below the subcorneal space (*Fuchs et al.*, 1977). The Na channels can be blocked by amiloride (N-amidino-3,5-diamino-6-chloropyrazine-carboxamide) added to the outer solution (e.g., *Cuthbert* and *Shum*, 1974). Na ions which have reached the cytosol $[(Na)_c]$ are then translocated into the interstitial space of the epithelium by pumps located

The authors wish to thank the Humboldt Foundation for supporting the stay of W.V.D. in Homburg and the Deutsche Forschungsgemeinschaft for supporting this work through SFB 38, project C1.

125

in the laterobasal membranes of the stratum granulosum and plasma membranes of deeper cell layers (e.g., *Cala, Cogswell* and *Mandel*, 1978). Pumping may occur partly in exchange for K. K ions taken up by the pump are returned to the interstitial space via passive, K-selective channels of the basolateral membranes. The cellular layers of the epithelium appear to be functionally coupled (e.g., *Rick et al.*, 1978). The paracellular shunt pathway of amphibian skin and urinary bladder can be relatively tight (high-resistance). (For a review of transport properties, see *Ussing, Erlij*, and *Lassen*, 1974; *Lindemann* and *Voûte*, 1976.)

SIMPLIFICATION THROUGH USE OF HIGH $(K)_i$

The high K-permeability of the inward-facing membranes should permit their depolarization by replacement of a large fraction of the interstitial Na by K (*Morel* and *Leblanc*, 1975). This substitution is expected to increase the membrane conductance about 4-fold (*Lindemann* and *Van Driessche*, 1978). The electrical properties of the epithelium will then be more nearly governed by those of the apical membrane, and the apical voltage will then be close to zero under overall short-circuit conditions. This will be particularly true when the apical resistance is kept large by using a low Na activity $[(Na)_o]$ in the outer solution and/or submaximal concentrations of amiloride. A further simplification can be achieved by using nonpenetrating anions like sulfate in all solutions.

STEADY-STATE SATURATION AND
MACROSCOPIC RELAXATION OF Na CURRENT

An interesting and widely investigated feature of Na translocation through the apical membrane is its saturation with increasing outer Na activity $[(Na)_o]$. The net Na current, as well as the membrane conductance and the unidirectional Na influx, increases only subproportionally with $(Na)_o$, thus resembling Michaelis-Menten kinetics. Concentration-step experiments with a fast-flow chamber have shown that when $(Na)_o$ is suddenly increased in exchange for K, the initial Na current flowing into the epithelium is considerably larger than the steady-state current. The transient current decreases to its steady-state value with a slow time course, taking several seconds (*Lindemann* and *Gebhardt*, 1973). The same relaxation phenomenon is observed while the inward-facing membranes are depolarized with higher $(K)_i$, i.e., while the apical membrane voltage presumably is close to zero. The decrease in current does not depend on an increase in $(Na)_c$. While the steady-state currents saturate, the peak transient currents show little or no saturation. Clearly, therefore, the membrane can pass transiently more Na current than its steady-state saturation curve would lead us to predict.

From these observations it was concluded that the translocating mechanism as such need not be easily saturable. It was suggested that saturation comes about by a $(Na)_o$-dependent and relatively slow decrease in the number of conducting translocators in the apical membrane (*Fuchs et al.*, 1977). The tenability of this hypothesis subsequently was investigated using noise analysis.

ORIGIN OF CURRENT FLUCTUATIONS

The activity of unsynchronized ion pumps is not expected to generate large current fluctuations because each pump unit transfers only a few charges per turnover cycle. However, by keeping $(Na)_c$ low, the pumps create a chemical Na gradient across the apical membrane. Therefore, it can be expected that possible fluctuations of Na current arising in the apical membrane will be diminished when the pump is blocked by ouabain. Thus, a decrease of current fluctuations observed after application of ouabain may not be taken as evidence that the fluctuations arose directly from the pump activity. Possible fluctuations arising from K-channels of inward-facing membranes are expected to be small if at high $(K)_i$ the electrochemical K gradient across these membranes is minimized. Current fluctuations arising in the paracellular shunt will be small when the shunt is tight. They are likely to be of the $1/f$ type and may then be recognized by this property. Thus, at high $(K)_i$ and high $(Na)_o$ the apical membrane will be the prime source of current fluctuations if its Na channels show spontaneous on-off kinetics or if such kinetics can be introduced with reversible blockers.

POWER DENSITY SPECTRA OF
SPONTANEOUS FLUCTUATIONS IN Na CURRENT

The macroscopic $(Na)_o$-dependent relaxation of Na current or Na permeability suggests that Na ions at the outer surface of the Na-selective membrane act as reversible blockers of Na channels. A simple model for this process would specify that transient binding of a Na ion to a receptor site can induce a conformational change which closes an adjacent Na channel for a mean time of several seconds. The Na channels would then show spontaneous on-off kinetics. The corresponding power density spectrum would be of the Lorentz type, with a corner frequency below 0.5 Hz. The current spectra actually obtained are in rough agreement with this expectation, particularly at frequencies above 0.5 Hz. However, their numerical evaluation is impeded by the fact that the plateau part of these "Lorentz curves," which is expected below 0.5 Hz, usually is not found to be horizontal, showing slopes between zero and −1 (*Lindemann* and *Van Driessche*, 1978). The same problem is apparent in voltage fluctuation spectra (*Segal*, 1972).

POWER DENSITY SPECTRA OBTAINED FROM AMILORIDE BLOCKAGE OF Na CHANNELS

Some quantitative information about the Na-translocation process can be obtained by the use of amiloride (*Lindemann* and *Van Driessche*, 1977a). As this drug is a reversible blocker of Na current, it may be expected to randomly interrupt the Na turnover of individual transport sites. Thus, in the presence of amiloride a site will either conduct fully or (when blocked) not conduct at all. The continuous current (i) passing one site is then chopped up into small current pulses of varying duration but equal amplitude (i). This use of reversible blockers may be of more general interest. It permits not only the computation of microscopic rate constants for the blocking process, but also the computation of turnover numbers and channel densities of the blocked translocators. Thus, even channels which do not show on-off kinetics of their own may be studied conveniently if a suitable blocker can be found.

The power density spectrum (PDS) of the amiloride-induced current fluctuations was found to approximate the Lorentz-type relatively closely. Amiloride rate constants could be computed from the dependence of corner frequency on amiloride concentration, a relationship which usually was found to be linear in the concentration range of 2-16 μM. The decrease of plateau power densities with amiloride concentration permitted the computation of the Na turnover at individual conducting translocators. At 60 mM sodium activity turnovers of more than 10^6 charges/sec were found. Therefore, it was inferred that transfer occurs through pores, these being the only high-rate translocators presently known (*Armstrong*, 1975). The density of amiloride-accessible pores (range 10^9/cm^2 in *Rana esculeuta*), as computed from the amiloride spectrum, was found to decrease when (Na)$_o$ was increased. This result was expected from our previous conclusion that Na blocks Na channels.

Na-DEPENDENCE OF CURRENT THROUGH OPEN PORES

The apical membrane can transiently pass more current than the saturating steady-state current-concentration curve indicates. As mentioned above, it was inferred from this observation that the current (i) through individual conducting translocators may not saturate in the (Na)$_o$ range where saturation of total Na current (I_{Na}) is already observed. Fluctuation analysis of the amiloride-modulated Na current provides the possibility to test this hypothesis further. To perform this test, amiloride-

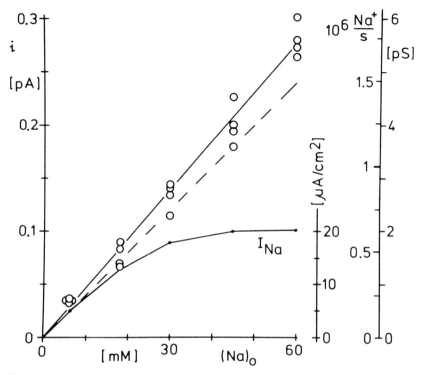

Fig. 1. Computed values of Na current (i) through single conducting pores at different outer Na activities. *Rana esculenta*, inner bathing solution high $(K)_i$. Data points are from one experiment; the dashed line represents mean values of 160 determinations of i in 9 experiments. Lower curve: saturation of macroscopic Na current. From *Lindemann* and *Van Driessche*, Proceedings of the International Union of Physiological Sciences XII:155, 1977.

induced current fluctuations were recorded at different $(Na)_o$ (*Lindemann and Van Driessche*, 1977b).

Figure 1 shows computed values of Na current (i) through single conducting pores obtained at different outer Na activities (abscissa). Amiloride concentrations between 1 and 16 μM could be used in this case. The dashed line represents the mean value of 160 determinations of i in 9 experiments. It appears that i, computed from amiloride spectra, increases linearly with $(Na)_o$. This result shows more directly that the saturation of the transport capacity of individual channels is not responsible for the saturation of the overall steady-state Na current observed in the same experiments (curve labeled I_{Na}). Thus, the saturation of I_{Na} may be accounted for by a decrease in the density of conducting pores with increasing $(Na)_o$.

REFERENCES

Armstrong, C.M.   1975.   Evidence for ionic pores in excitable membranes. Biophys J 15:932–933

Cala, P.M., Cogswell, N., and Mandel, L.J.   1978.   Binding of ^{3}H-ouabain to split frog skin. The role of the Na-K ATPase in the generation of short circuit current. J Gen Physiol 71:347–367

Cuthbert, A.W., and Shum, W.K.   1974.   Amiloride and the sodium channel. Arch Pharmacol 281:261–269

Fuchs, W., Hviid Larsen, E., and Lindemann, B.   1977.   Current voltage curve of sodium channels and concentration dependence of sodium permeability in frog skin. J Physiol (Lond) 267:137–166

Higgins, J.T., Gebler, B., and Frömter, E.   1977.   Electrical properties of amphibian urinary bladder epithelia. II. The cell potential profile in *Necturus maculosus*. Pflüg Arch 371:87–97

Koefoed-Johnsen, V., and Ussing, H.H.   1958.   The nature of the frog skin potential. Acta Physiol Scand 42:298–308

Leaf, A.   1965.   Transepithelial transport and its hormonal control in the toad bladder. Ergebn Physiol 56:216–263

Lindemann, B., and Gebhardt, U.   1973.   Delayed changes of Na-permeability in response to steps of (Na) at the outer surface of frog skin and frog bladder. In *Transport Mechanisms in Epithelia*, ed. H.H. Ussing and N.A. Thorn, pp. 115–130., Copenhagen: Munksgaard

Lindemann, B., and Van Driessche, W.   1977a.   Sodium specific membrane channels of frog skin are pores: Current fluctuations reveal high turnover. Science 195:292–294

Lindemann, B., and Van Driessche, W.   1977b.   Mechanism of sodium-uptake through the sodium-selective membrane of frog skin epithelium. Proceedings of the Internat. Union of Physiological Sciences, XII:155

Lindemann, B., and Van Driessche, W.   1978.   The Mechanism of Na-uptake through Na-selective channels in the epithelium of frog skin. In *Membrane Transport Processes*, Vol. 1, ed. by J.F. Hoffman, pp. 155–178. New York: Raven Press

Lindemann, B., and Voûte, C.   1976.   Structure and Function of the Epidermis. In *Frog Neurobiology*, ed. R. Llinás and W. Precht, pp. 169–210. Berlin-New York: Springer Verlag

Morel, F., and Leblanc, G.   1975.   Transient current changes and Na compartmentalization in frog skin epithelium. Pflüg Arch 358:135–157

Nagel, W.   1977.   The dependence of the electrical potentials across the membranes of the frog skin upon the concentration of sodium in the mucosal solution. J Physiol (Lond.) 269:777–796

Rick, R., Dörge, A., von Arnim, E., and Thurau, K.   1978.   Electron microprobe analysis of frog skin epithelium: evidence for a syncytial sodium transport compartment. J Membr Biol 39:313–331

Segal, J.R.   1972.   Electrical fluctuations associated with active transport. Biophys J 12:1371–1390

Ussing, H.H., Erlij, D., and Lassen, U.   1974.   Transport pathways in biological membranes. Ann Rev Physiol 36:17–49

Ussing, H.H., and Windhager, E.E.   1964.   Nature of shunt path and active sodium transport path through frog skin epithelium. Acta Physiol Scand 62:484–504

Amiloride and Epithelial Sodium Transport
Edited by A.W. Cuthbert, G.M. Fanelli, Jr. and A. Scriabine

Onset of Amiloride Sensitivity in the Developing Pig Colon

M. W. Smith, D. Cremaschi**, D. R. Ferguson‡,
S. Hénin†, P. S. James* and G. Meyer†*

**ARC Institute of Animal Physiology
Babraham, Cambridge, U.K.
** Istituto di Fisiologia Generale
Universita di Baria
Via Amendola 165/A, Bari, Italy
† Istituto di Fisiologia Generale e di Chimica Biologica
Universita di Milano
Via Mangiagalli, 32, Italy
‡ Department of Pharmacology
University of Cambridge
Cambridge, U.K.*

The newborn pig acquires a passive immunity to disease by the intestinal absorption of ingested immunoglobulins. This process involves the endocytosis of large quantities of intact protein and the formation of protein-containing vacuoles within the cell cytoplasm. Vacuoles increase in size as protein transport continues, causing considerable distortion of the whole mucosa. The ability of the intestine to absorb nutrients was observed to be reduced under these circumstances (*Henriques de Jesus* and *Smith*, 1974a,b), but nothing was known about the functioning of the colon during early development. Initial experiments, carried out on the proximal colon *in vitro*, showed it to transport methionine from lumen to blood via a process similar to that seen in the small intestine of adult animals (*James* and *Smith*, 1976; *Hénin* and *Smith*, 1976). It is now known that the proximal region of the neonatal colon can actively transport a wide variety of neutral amino acids. Lipid droplets also appear in the mucosal cells of the proximal colon in the 1-day-old animal, suggesting that lipid absorption takes place *in vivo* during early development (*Bentley* and *Smith*, 1975). These unusual properties may allow the pig to

This work was supported by NATO grant 1429.

Table 1.   Unidirectional Na Fluxes Measured Across Short-circuited Preparations of Distal Colon Taken from Newborn and 1-day-old Pigs

Age (days)	Na Transport (μEq cm^{-2} hr^{-1})			Short-circuit Current (μA cm^{-2})
	Influx	Efflux	Net flux	
0	7.20 ± 1.09	3.10 ± 0.35	4.10	61 ± 8.0
1	11.9 ± 0.97	3.50 ± 1.26	8.40	112 ± 21.0

Values represent means ± SE of five determinations in each case.
Data from *Bentley* and *Smith* (1975).

maintain efficient absorption of nutrients at a time when the small intestine is mainly concerned with the absorption of immunoglobulins.

The distal colon transports neither amino acids nor lipids, but it does transport Na by a process which changes during early development. Results of *Bentley* and *Smith* (1975), showing time-dependent changes in Na transport in the distal colon, are summarized in Table 1. Both the net flux of Na and the short-circuit current double during the first 24 hours of postnatal life. The increase in net flux is completely accounted for by a corresponding increase in the mucosa-to-serosa flux of Na. It should be pointed out, however, that although the short-circuit current increases in parallel with the net flux of Na, its value is always considerably less than would be expected if Na were the only ion to be actively transported by this tissue. The initial objective of the present work was to follow these changes in Na transport and short-circuit current during the first 10 days of postnatal life. It soon became obvious, however, that the tissue sensitivity to amiloride also changed during this early period of development. It was then decided to relate these changes to the other measurements of Na transport.

COLONIC SHORT-CIRCUIT CURRENT
MEASURED DURING EARLY POSTNATAL DEVELOPMENT

Pieces of distal colon clamped in Ussing-type chambers were bathed at 37°C in glucose-free bicarbonate medium (*Krebs* and *Henseleit*, 1932) gassed with a mixture of 95% O_2 and 5% CO_2. Figure 1 shows the short-circuit current measured across these preparations after approximately 10 min incubation. The absolute short-circuit current showed a sixfold increase during the first 10 days of postnatal life. Amiloride, present at a concentration of 5×10^{-6} M in the mucosal solution, had no effect on the short-circuit current of newborn pig colon (85 ± 7.7 and 79.5 ± 7.5 μA cm^{-2} for control and amiloride-treated colons, respectively, 20 observations). Amiloride did, however, partially block the short-circuit current of distal colons taken from older animals, the amiloride-sensitive current increasing from 70 to 390 μA cm^{-2} from day 1 to day 9 of postnatal life.

There was always a part of the short-circuit current which remained resistant to inhibition by amiloride. This remained constant, at about 75 μA cm^{-2}, during the first week of postnatal life, but it showed a significant increase in colons taken from 9-day-old animals (160 μA cm^{-2}; difference from the newborn colon statistically significant at the 0.001 level of probability).

The sensitivity of the distal colon to different concentrations of amiloride was tested in another series of experiments. The results obtained are shown in Figure 2. The minimal concentration of amiloride

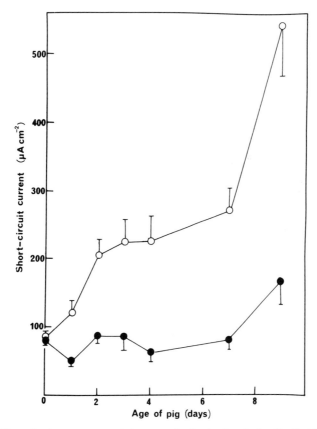

Fig. 1. Short-circuit current recorded across pig distal colon during the first 10 days of postnatal development. Tissues were incubated in bicarbonate saline and the short-circuit current recorded in the absence (O) and presence (●) of 5 × 10^{-6}M amiloride. Values give the mean short-circuit current ± SE of between 4–20 paired comparisons.

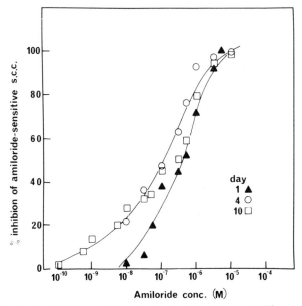

Fig. 2. Amiloride inhibition of pig colonic short-circuit current. The concentration of amiloride in the mucosal solution was increased, by stepwise addition of amiloride, until there was no further decrease in short-circuit current. This is then referred to as 100% inhibition and the effect of lower concentrations of amiloride is related to this value. Distal colons were taken from pigs on days 1 (▲), 4 (○) and 10 (□). Each value gives the mean of at least five determinations.

needed to produce an inhibitory effect on short-circuit current depended on the age of the pig (i.e., about 10^{-9} M for 4- and 10-day-old pigs, and about 2×10^{-8} M for the 1-day-old animal). The amiloride-sensitive sites in the 1-day-old pig colon may have properties different from those seen in older animals. The presence of amiloride at a concentration of 2.5×10^{-6} M, however, causes maximal inhibition in all cases.

Further information on the action of amiloride, i.e., whether it blocks electrogenic Na entry and, if so, whether this pathway can contribute significantly to brush-border membrane conductance, can be obtained by recording intracellular membrane potentials under different experimental conditions. These experiments were confined to distal colons taken from 0- and 4-day-old animals. The microelectrodes used had tip resistances of the order of 30 MΩ and tip potentials of less than 5 mV. They were inserted into cells from the luminal side and the membrane potentials recorded, using conventional techniques, taking the mucosal solution as zero potential. Transmural potentials were recorded using calomel half-cells connected to the mucosal and serosal solutions through agar bridges containing 3 M KCl. The ratio R_m/R_s (microvillar membrane resistance/basolateral membrane resistance) was determined by passing 150 μA cm^{-2} in 1-sec pulses across the tissue, while at the same time recording the drop in voltage across both microvillar and basolateral membranes. Alternate current pulses had opposite polarity to avoid polarization of the cell membranes. The results obtained for the two ages of colon are shown in Figure 3.

The microvillar membrane potential of distal colons taken from newborn pigs remained unaffected by the presence of amiloride (-45.8 ± 0.7, -46.0 ± 0.6 and -46.8 ± 0.9 mV, before, during and after the application of 2.5×10^{-6} M amiloride, respectively). The transmural potential remained constant at about 5 mV throughout these experiments

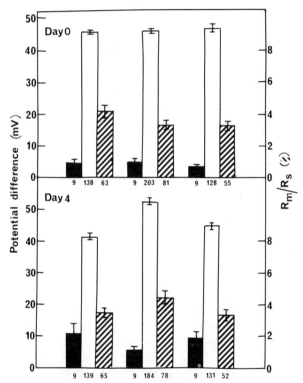

Fig. 3.   Effect of amiloride on microvillar membrane potential (V_m), transmural potential (V_{ms}) and cell membrane resistance ratio (R_m/R_s) measured using distal colons taken from newborn and 4-day-old pigs. The concentration of amiloride used was 2.5×10^{-6} M. Electrical parameters were first measured over a period of 30 min. Amiloride was then added to the mucosal solution and the measurements repeated for a further 30-min period. Amiloride was then removed and the measurements continued for a final 30-min period. Numbers represent the number of observations on which mean values $\pm$ SE are based. Nine pigs from each age group were used for these experiments. ■ and □ represent V_{ms} and V_m, respectively; ▨ represents R_m/R_s.

and there was no significant change in the R_m/R_s ratio. The microvillar membrane potential of distal colons taken from 4-day-old pigs was significantly less than that found in the newborn animal (-40.7 ± 1.0 compared with -45.8 ± 0.7 mV, $P < 0.001$). Addition of amiloride caused a significant hyperpolarization of the microvillar membrane potential in the 4-day-old pig colon (from -40.7 ± 1.0 to -52.2 ± 0.8 mV, $P < 0.001$) and a fall in transmural potential from 10.2 ± 2.8 to 5.5 ± 1.2 mV. The R_m/R_s ratio, calculated from the two control periods of measurement, was increased in the presence of amiloride (1.68 ± 0.12 to 2.20 ± 0.23, $P < 0.05$). All these effects were completely reversible.

The age-dependent decrease in the microvillar membrane potential could reflect an increased Na permeability across this membrane. The hyperpolarization seen in the 4-day-old colon in the presence of amiloride, the fall in transmural potential and the increase in the R_m/R_s ratio are all similar to effects recorded previously using colons taken from adult rabbits (*Schultz, Frizzell*, and *Nellans*, 1977). All these effects are induced in the pig colon during the first four days of postnatal life.

If amiloride does reduce the Na permeability of the microvillar membrane of the 4-day-old pig colon, one might predict that this would affect the Na content of the mucosal tissue. This was tested for in a further series of experiments. Pieces of distal colon, taken from 0- and 4-day-old piglets, were incubated as everted sacs in bicarbonate medium. [³H] PEG-900 was added to the serosal solution for a period of 45 min for subsequent measurement of extracellular space. The mucosa was then scraped and weighed and the cells disrupted by freezing and boiling in distilled water. Sodium was determined by flame photometry and a correction applied for fluid left in contact with the microvillar surface of the incubated colons. In some experiments ²²Na was added to the mucosal solution 15 min before scraping the mucosa to determine radiochemically the rapidly exchangeable pool of Na within the colonic mucosa. The results obtained are shown in Table 2.

The overall concentration of Na in pig colonic mucosa was not changed by development or by the presence of amiloride. The radiochemically determined Na concentration was similarly unaffected by development, but amiloride reduced this rapidly exchangeable Na pool by about 40%. The fact that the total Na shows no change but the radiochemically determined Na concentration does change with amiloride suggests that the Na transport pool represents only a small fraction of the total Na present. This is consistent with results obtained previously using rabbit colon where electrophysiological measurements suggested a Na transport pool of about 14 mM (*Schultz, Frizzell*, and *Nellans*, 1977).

Table 2. Effect of Amiloride on Intramucosal Na Concentrations Determined in Distal Colons from Newborn and 4-day-old Pigs

	Mucosal Na Concentration (mM)			
	Newborn		4-day-old	
	Na	Na*	Na	Na*
Control	80.9 ± 4.1	42.3 ± 5.8	89.4 ± 5.0	35.0 ± 2.5
	(12)	(4)	(13)	(6)
Amiloride	71.6 ± 6.0	38.3 ± 3.4	78.9 ± 6.0	22.1 ± 2.1
(2.5×10^{-6} M)	(10)	(4)	(14)	(6)
P	n.s.	n.s.	n.s.	<0.02

Incubation conditions were as stated in text. Na and Na* refer to chemically and radiochemically determined Na concentrations within the pig colonic mucosa. Number of determinations given in parentheses.

The situation at birth, when amiloride has no effect on short-circuit current, changes in four days to one where a large proportion of the short-circuit current becomes sensitive to amiloride. The way in which amiloride produces its effect on the 4-day-old pig colon appears, superficially, to resemble that recorded previously for other colons taken from adult animals (*Frizzell, Koch*, and *Schultz*, 1976; *Yorio* and *Bentley*, 1977; *Dawson*, 1977; *Schultz, Frizzell*, and *Nellans*, 1977). It must be remembered, however, that these results only apply to measurements of short-circuit current and that short-circuit is *not* equivalent to net Na transport in the neonatal pig colon.

Results summarized in Table 3 show that this non-correspondence between Na transport and short-circuit current in the large intestine applies to several species. It is only in the frog and rabbit that the short-circuit current can be fully accounted for by the net transport of Na. Even when correspondence is good, one can still find a small but statistically significant short-circuit current resistant to high concentrations of amiloride (*Frizzell, Koch*, and *Schultz*, 1976, using 10^{-4} M amiloride). For these reasons, it seemed prudent to repeat work on the neontal pig colon, making direct measurements of Na flux. These experiments form the basis of the second part of this paper.

SODIUM FLUXES MEASURED ACROSS DISTAL PIG COLON DURING EARLY POSTNATAL DEVELOPMENT

Both unidirectional (^{22}Na) and bidirectional (^{24}Na mucosa-to-serosa; ^{22}Na serosa-to-mucosa) fluxes were measured across short-circuited

Table 3.   Degree of Correspondence between Short-circuit Currents Measured Across Different *In Vitro* Preparations of Large Intestine and Their Respective Net Na Fluxes

Species	Short-circuit Current (μA cm^{-2})		% Correspondence	Source
	Measured	Calculated from Net Na Flux		
Turtle	73	60	81	*Dawson*, 1977
Frog	107	98	92	*Cooperstein* and *Hogben*, 1959
Rabbit	77	76	99	*Frizzell, Koch*, and *Schultz*, 1976
Rabbit	80	88	110	*Yorio* and *Bentley*, 1977
Human	86	107	124	*Grady, Duhamel*, and *Moore*, 1970
Human	187	271	145	*Archampong, Harris*, and *Clark*, 1972
Piglet				
(day 0)	61	110	180	*Bentley* and *Smith*, 1975
(day 1)	112	225	201	
Rat				
(stripped)	27	129	480	*Binder* and *Rawlins*, 1973
(unstripped)	37	240	737	

The calculated short-circuit currents are computed assuming that Na is the only ion to be actively transported across the epithelium.

preparations of distal colon taken from pigs during the first 10 days of postnatal development. The results are summarized in Table 4. The backflux of Na remained constant throughout early development (overall mean, 3.9 μEq cm^{-2} hr^{-1}). The influx of Na doubled during the first 24 hours of postnatal life, giving over a twofold increase in net flux. There was no further increase in influx during development, so the net flux of Na then remained reasonably constant. This is in contrast to the short-circuit current which had been shown previously to increase in a more or less linear fashion throughout the first 10 days of postnatal life (Fig. 1).

These experiments on Na flux were next repeated in the presence of 5×10^{-6} M amiloride. The net fluxes of Na measured under these conditions are compared with those for control tissues in Figure 4. The presence of amiloride had no effect on the net transport of Na across the colon of the newborn animal. The fall in amiloride-insensitive net Na flux, seen using colons of 1-day-old animals, is probably significant; however, it is not possible to be sure of this, since most of the work involved measuring unidirectional rather than bidirectional fluxes of Na. The amiloride-insensitive net Na flux, measured at later times in development, appeared to be roughly constant at about 2 μEq cm^{-2} hr^{-1}. This represented about one-third of the net Na flux measured under control conditions.

We have as yet no firm idea as to how this Na crosses the colon. It could represent a neutral transport of NaCl or NaHCO$_3$ (there is a net Cl flux across the short-circuited *proximal* colon of the 1-day-old pig of the order of 1 μEq cm^{-2} hr^{-1}; *Bentley* and *Smith*, 1975), or it could be that part of the colonic transport of Na occurs by an amiloride-resistant pathway similar to that found in the small intestine. It is interesting to note, for instance, that the amiloride-resistant short-circuit current is roughly equivalent to the amiloride-resistant Na transport in colons taken from these older animals.

RELATION BETWEEN AMILORIDE-SENSITIVE Na FLUX AND AMILORIDE-SENSITIVE SHORT-CIRCUIT CURRENT MEASURED DURING EARLY DEVELOPMENT

The measurements of short-circuit current showing an increase in amiloride-sensitive current during the first nine days of postnatal life (illustrated in Figure 1) were made within 10 min of setting up each preparation. They are not directly comparable to measurements of net

Table 4. Sodium Fluxes Measured Across Short-circuited Preparations of Distal Colons Taken from Pigs During the First 10 days of Postnatal Development

Time (days)	Na Transport (μEq cm^{-2} hr^{-1})		
	Influx	Efflux	Net flux
0	7.64 ± 0.83 (15)	3.86 ± 0.37 (13)	3.78
1	13.80 ± 0.98 (8)	4.47 ± 1.09 (8)	9.33
4	10.10 ± 1.4 (6)	3.66 ± 0.73 (6)	6.44
7	12.40 ± 0.89 (4)	4.0 ± 0.55 (4)	8.40
10	10.60 ± 1.8 (5)	3.34 ± 0.89 (5)	7.26

Conditions of incubation were as described by *Bentley* and *Smith*, 1975, but without glucose in the incubation medium. Values represent means ± SE, with the number of determinations given in parentheses.

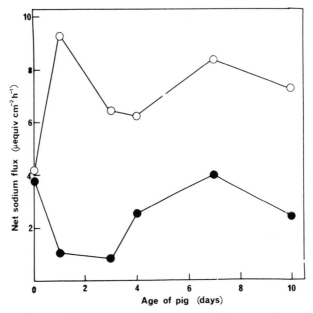

Fig. 4. Net fluxes of Na measured across short-circuited preparations of distal colon taken from pigs of different ages. Experiments were carried out in the absence (O) and presence (●) of 5×10^{-6} M amiloride. Each value is derived from 4–15 separate determinations of Na influx and efflux.

Na flux carried out under steady-state conditions. Direct comparisons can be made, however, using currents measured over time periods identical to those used for Na flux measurements. These amiloride-sensitive short-circuit currents can then be converted to μEq Na cm^{-2} hr^{-1}, again assuming that Na is the only ion to be actively transported. In Figure 5 these results are compared with the amiloride-sensitive net flux of Na.

The distal colon of the newborn pig shows no amiloride-sensitive Na transport and no amiloride-sensitive short-circuit current. The amiloride-sensitive current increases only slightly during the first 24 hr of postnatal development, but there is a big increase in amiloride-sensitive Na transport. This results in a sevenfold discrepancy between amiloride-sensitive Na fluxes calculated by the two different methods. This discrepancy is gradually reduced as development continues, and by nine days there is good agreement between these two measurements. The colonic epithelium of the neonatal pig is replaced over a period of four days (*Jarvis et al.*, 1977), so that the initial increase in the amiloride sensitivity of the directly determined Na flux, seen one day after birth, must occur within the epithelial layer which was present at birth. Already there is evidence suggesting that the nature of the amiloride-sensitive sites appearing at this time is different from that seen in older animals (Fig. 2). Our present hypothesis is that amiloride inhibits the neutral entry of NaCl in the 1-day-old pig colon. We are presently in the process of testing this hypothesis further.

POSSIBLE CAUSE OF DEVELOPING AMILORIDE SENSITIVITY IN PIG DISTAL COLON

Developmental changes in intestinal function arise primarily from alterations in a cell's environment. This environment consists of the intestinal lumen as well as the blood. A change in the composition of either could have important effects on transport. Ileostomies were therefore performed on a number of newborn pigs to test whether the luminal environment is important for the induction of developmental changes in Na

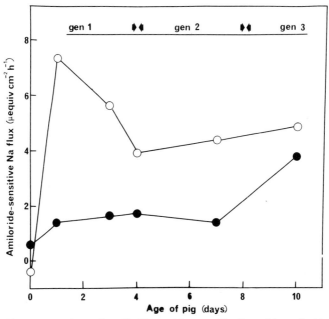

Fig. 5. Direct comparison of amiloride-sensitive net Na flux with amiloride-sensitive short-circuit current measured across distal colons taken from pigs during early postnatal development. Amiloride-sensitive Na fluxes were either measured isotopically (O) or calculated assuming the amiloride-sensitive short-circuit current to represent the electrogenic transport of Na (●). The numbers 1, 2 and 3 across top of figure refer to the first, second and third generations of colonic epithelial cells.

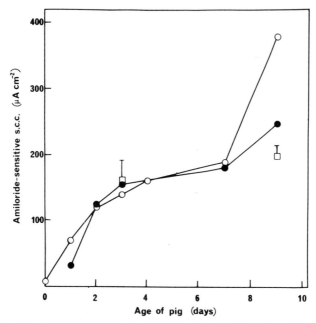

Fig. 6.   Effect of ileostomy on the development of amiloride-sensitive short-circuit current measured across the distal colons of neonatal pigs. Ileostomies were performed on newborn pigs which were then killed 3 and 9 days later. Short-circuit currents were measured in the presence and absence of 5×10^{-6} M amiloride. The amiloride-sensitive currents measured across colons taken from ileostomized pigs (□) were then compared with those found in control (O) and sham-operated (●) animals. Values for ileostomized pigs represent means ± SE of determinations carried out on four different pieces of tissue.

transport. Other newborn pigs were subjected to a sham operation technique. Piglets were returned to the sow immediately after recovery from the anesthetic, to be killed at known times afterwards. The amiloride sensitivity of short-circuit current was measured across the distal colons of these animals and the results compared with those found previously in a control situation. The results obtained are shown in Figure 6. The time course for onset of amiloride sensitivity of short-circuit current was not affected by sham operation or by ileostomy. The piglets were fed normally following these operative techniques. It was concluded from these experiments that it is not necessary for food to pass along the lumen of the colon for changes in Na transport to take place. Some of these results have already been published in preliminary form (*James* and *Smith*, 1977).

Aldosterone is known to induce changes in Na transport across high-resistance epithelia, and it has been shown that these changes are associated with an increase in the number of amiloride-sensitive Na sites present (*Cuthbert, Okpako,* and *Shum,* 1974; *Cuthbert* and *Shum,* 1976). Preliminary measurements of aldosterone in the blood serum of neonatal pigs show the level to increase shortly after birth (*J.Y.F. Paterson,* unpublished results). The injection of potassium 17β hydroxy-3-oxo-17α-pregna-4,6-diene-21-carboxylate (Soludactone®), an inhibitor of aldosterone action, abolishes the time-dependent increase in amiloride-sensitive short-circuit current. These results suggest that aldosterone is responsible for at least some of the changes in Na transport taking place during development. This possibility is being investigated further at the present time.

REFERENCES

Archampong, E.Q., Harris, J., and Clark, C.G. 1972. The absorption and secretion of water and electrolytes across the healthy and diseased human colonic mucosa measured *in vitro.* Gut 13:880–886

Bentley, P.J. and Smith, M.W. 1975. Transport of electrolytes across the helicoidal colon of the new-born pig. J Physiol (Lond.) 249:103–117

Binder H.J. and Rawlins, C.L. 1973. Electrolyte transport across isolated large intestinal mucosa. Am J Physiol, 225:1232–1239

Cooperstein, I.L. and Hogben, C.A. 1959. Ionic transfer across the isolated frog large intestine. J Gen Physiol 42:461–473

Cuthbert, A.W., Okpako, D. and Shum, W.K. 1974. Aldosterone and the number of sodium channels in frog skin. Br J Pharmac 51:128–129P

Cuthbert, A.W. and Shum, W.K. 1976. Estimation of the lifespan of amiloride binding sites in the membranes of toad bladder epithelial cells. J Physiol (Lond) 255:605–618

Dawson, D.C. 1977. Na and Cl transport across the isolated turtle colon: parallel pathways for transmural ion movement. J Membr Biol 37:213–233

Frizzell, R.A., Koch, M.J. and Schultz, S.G. 1976. Ion transport by rabbit colon. I. Active and passive components. J Membr Biol 27:297–316

Grady, G.F., Duhamel, R.C. and Moore, E.W. 1970. Active transport of sodium by human colon *in vitro.* Gastroenterology 59:583–588

Hénin, S. and Smith, M.W. 1976. Electrical properties of pig colonic mucosa measured during early post-natal development. J Physiol (Lond) 262:169–187

Henriques de Jesus, C. and Smith, M.W. 1974a. Sodium transport by the small intestine of new-born and suckling pigs. J Physiol (Lond) 243:211–224

Henriques de Jesus, C. and Smith, M.W. 1974b. Protein and glucose induced changes in sodium transport across the pig small intestine. J Physiol (Lond) 243:225–242

James, P.S. and Smith, M.W. 1976. Methionine transport by pig colonic mucosa measured during early post-natal development. J Physiol (Lond) 262:151–168

James, P.S. and Smith, M.W. 1977. Effect of ileostomy on changing transport function in the new-born pig colon. J Physiol (Lond) 272:61–62P

Jarvis, L.G., Morgan, G., Smith, M.W. and Wooding, F.B.P. 1977. Cell replacement and changing transport function in the neonatal pig colon. J Physiol (Lond) 273:717-729

Krebs, H.A. and Henseleit, K. 1932. Untersuchungen über die Harnstoff-bildung im Tierkörper. Hoppe-Seyler's Z. Physiol Chem 210:33–66

Schultz, S.G., Frizzell, R.A. and Nellans, H.N. 1977. Active sodium transport and the electrophysiology of rabbit colon. J Membr Biol 33:351–384

Yorio, T. and Bentley, P.J. 1977. Permeability of the rabbit colon in vitro. Am J Physiol 232:F5–F9

© 1979 Urban & Schwarzenberg, Inc. Baltimore-Munich
Amiloride and Epithelial Sodium Transport
Edited by A.W. Cuthbert, G.M. Fanelli, Jr. and A. Scriabine

Autoregulation of Amiloride-Sensitive Sodium Entry in Mammalian Colon

Raymond A. Frizzell

Department of Physiology
University of Pittsburgh
School of Medicine
Pittsburgh, Pennsylvania 15261

Descending rabbit colon, when studied *in vitro*, displays several properties normally associated with Na-transporting epithelia: a) The transepithelial electrical potential difference (ψ_{ms}) and short-circuit current (I_{sc}) are entirely attributable to the rate of active Na absorption from mucosa to serosa (*Frizzell, Koch*, and *Schultz*, 1976); b) amiloride abolishes Na transport by inhibiting Na entry from the mucosal solution into the transporting cells (*Frizzell* and *Turnheim*, 1978); and c) aldosterone elicits equivalent increases in I_{sc} and the rate of Na absorption (*Frizzell* and *Schultz*, 1978). Although this tissue also actively absorbs Cl, the Cl transport process appears to be electrically silent and most likely involves a neutral exchange with HCO_3 which is secreted by mammalian colon (*Frizzell et al.*, 1976; *Phillips* and *Schmalz*, 1970; *Schultz, Frizzell*, and *Nellans*, 1977).

More recent studies suggest that Na entry into the transporting cells via the amiloride-sensitive pathway is normally the rate-limiting step in transepithelial Na transport, and that variations in the rate of Na absorption by this tissue appear to be determined by changes in mucosal membrane permeability to Na.

a) Spontaneous variations in the rate of Na absorption (J^{Na}_{net}) are highly correlated with variations in the rate of Na entry across the mucosal

Research support derived from the U.S.P.H.S., NIH grants AM-16275 and AM-18199 (NIAMDD), the Western Pennsylvania Heart Association, and the Wechsler Research Foundation. The author is supported by a NIH Research Career Development Award (AM-00173).

membrane (J_{mc}^{Na}) in a one-for-one fashion (*Frizzell* and *Turnheim*, 1978)

b) Amphotericin B, added to the mucosal solution, has no effect on I_{sc} or J_{net}^{Na} of tissues spontaneously absorbing Na at rates of approximately 5 μEq/cm²hr, but increases the I_{sc} of tissues absorbing at lower rates to this value (*Frizzell* and *Turnheim*, 1978). Amphotericin always increases tissue conductance (G_t) and J_{mc}^{Na} regardless of whether it affects I_{sc} or J_{net}^{Na}; thus, the effects of this agent appear to be due to the formation of pathways for Na entry across the mucosal membrane which parallel the normal amiloride-sensitive entry paths.

c) Certain sulfonated anions (e.g., isethionate) stimulate *amiloride-sensitive* Na entry across the mucosal membrane and may elicit a "maximal" rate of Na absorption similar to that produced by amphotericin (*Turnheim, Frizzell* and *Schultz*, 1977). If J_{net}^{Na} is elevated to the maximal rate with isethionate, amphotericin has no additional effect on the I_{sc}.

d) Aldosterone stimulates a "maximal" rate of Na absorption (approximately 5 μEq/cm²hr) and subsequent addition of amphotericin has no further effect on J_{net}^{Na} (*Frizzell* and *Schultz*, 1978).

All of these findings suggest that maximal spontaneous or induced rates of Na transport reflect a saturation of the Na pump mechanism at the basolateral membranes so that Na extrusion from the cell to the serosal solution becomes the rate-limiting step in transepithelial Na transport.

The effects of stimulatory anions in this regard are particularly interesting. A direct correlation is observed between the extent to which these anions increase the I_{sc} and the simultaneous increase in tissue conductance which they elicit (*Turnheim et al.*, 1977). This increase in G_t is attributable to an increase in the conductance of the amiloride-sensitive Na entry step. There is no tendency toward saturation of I_{sc} with increasing G_t, as is observed with amphotericin (*Frizzell* and *Turnheim*, 1978); anions only increase tissue conductance if they also increase the rate of Na absorption. This observation implies that when Na transport is elevated to the maximal level by increasing the conductance of the amiloride-sensitive pathway, a further increase in the conductance of this pathway cannot be elicited, i.e., a maximal pump rate precludes additional Na entry into the cell, suggesting a feedback interaction between the pump rate and the permeability of the amiloride-sensitive Na entry step.

Several observations obtained from other Na-transporting epithelia are in accord with a feedback mechanism of this type. In 1961 *MacRob-*

bie and *Ussing* concluded that inhibition of the Na pump in frog skin with ouabain led to a decrease in the Na permeability of the outer membrane. Subsequently, other investigators, using more direct approaches, found that impaired pump activity led to a decreased rate of Na entry (or increased electrical resistance) across the outer or mucosal membranes of frog or toad skin (*Biber*, 1971; *Larsen*, 1973; *Erlij* and *Smith*, 1973; *Moreno et al.*, 1973; *Rick, Dürge,* and *Nagel,* 1975; *Helman* and *Nagel,* 1977) and toad (*Essig* and *Leaf,* 1963; *Finn,* 1975) and rabbit (*Lewis, Eaton,* and *Diamond,* 1976) urinary bladder. In addition, *Cuthbert* and *Shum* (1977) have recently demonstrated that inhibition of the Na pump in frog skin decreased the number of specific amiloride-binding sites at the outer membranes. Since a reduction in the rate of Na extrusion across the basolateral membrane will result in an increased intracellular Na concentration, it is reasonable to suggest that cell Na may serve as the negative feedback effector which decreases the permeability of the outer or mucosal membrane to Na.[1]

Several additional findings obtained using isolated rabbit colon are consistent with this view (*Turnheim, Frizzell,* and *Schultz,* 1978). When the I_{sc} is abolished by ouabain, a decrease in tissue conductance is also observed, whose magnitude is equal to the amiloride-sensitive component of G_t (i.e., equal to the conductance of the active Na transport pathway, $_aG_{Na}$). Following ouabain inhibition of the I_{sc}, amiloride has no further effect on tissue conductance, suggesting that $_aG_{Na}$ was abolished by ouabain. The results presented in Table 1 indicate that the effect of ouabain on $_aG_{Na}$ is due to a decrease in the conductance of the Na entry step. Ouabain decreases Na entry across the mucosal membranes of rabbit colon; the reduction in J_{me}^{Na} (unidirectional Na influx from the mucosal solution into the epithelium) does not differ significantly from the decline in I_{sc} produced by the glycoside. The remainder of J_{me}^{Na} represents Na entry into the paracellular pathways (*Frizzell* and *Turnheim,* 1978).

Exposure of the mucosal surface of rabbit colon to amphotericin also may increase cellular Na levels since this agent enhances Na entry into the cells and elicits a maximal rate of Na absorption (*Frizzell* and *Turnheim,* 1978). The effect of amiloride on I_{sc}, G_t and J_{me}^{Na} in tissues exposed to amphotericin also is given in Table 1. The maximal I_{sc} elicited by amphotericin in these experiments is 4 μEq/cm^{2}hr. Under these conditions, amiloride has no effect on I_{sc}, G_t or J_{me}^{Na}.

[1] Although the experiments described here were intended to elucidate the effects of changes in $[Na]_c$ on mucosal membrane Na permeability, reciprocal changes in $[K]_c$ undoubtedly accompany many of these manipulations. Therefore, the possibility that changes in $[K]_c$ (or the activities of other intracellular ions) are responsible for these observations, as postulated by *Robinson* and *Macknight* (1976), cannot be excluded.

Table 1. Effects of Ouabain, Amphotericin and Amiloride on Unidirectional Na Influx (J_{me}^{Na})

	G_t	I_{sc}	J_{me}^{Na}
Control (20)	4.5 ± 0.2	1.5 ± 0.2	3.1 ± 0.2
+ Ouabain	$3.8 \pm 0.2^*$	$0.1 \pm 0.1^*$	$1.8 \pm 0.1^*$
Amphotericin (16)	4.8 ± 0.4	4.0 ± 0.2	6.3 ± 0.2
+ Amiloride	5.1 ± 0.4	4.0 ± 0.3	6.3 ± 0.4

Values of I_{sc} and J_{me}^{Na} in $\mu Eq/cm^2hr$; G_t in mmhos/cm². Ouabain, 10^{-4} M; amphotericin, 15 $\mu g/ml$; amiloride, 10^{-4} M. Data for each pair of observations were obtained using tissues from the same animal; number of paired determinations given in parentheses.

* Significant difference from corresponding control value.

Thus, both ouabain and amphotericin abolish the amiloride-sensitive components of G_t and J_{me}^{Na}. In the case of amphotericin, one might argue that the normal, amiloride-sensitive pathway is simply overshadowed by the formation of parallel channels for Na entry into the cell. However, under normal conditions, the amiloride-sensitive component of J_{me}^{Na} averages 2–2.5 $\mu Eq/cm^2hr$; thus, the presence of this component should have resulted in a 30–40% reduction in J_{me}^{Na} by amiloride, which would be readily detectable. Thus, as discussed above, the effects of ouabain and amphotericin on $_aG_{Na}$ and J_{me}^{Na} appear to be mediated by an increase in the intracellular Na pool which abolishes the normal Na entry step.

Figure 1 illustrates the effect on amiloride-sensitive I_{sc} (plotted as I_{Na}^m) of exposure of rabbit colon to a sudden increase in the Na concentration of the bathing media at zero-time. In these experiments tissues were preincubated in Na-free media for 30–45 min so that the amiloride-sensitive current was abolished and the tissue was depleted of Na. Following addition of 140 mM Na to the bathing media, the Na current across the mucosal membrane, I_{Na}^m, undergoes a transient overshoot which then declines to a steady-state level of 2 $\mu Eq/cm^2hr$. Similar findings have been reported by *Morel* and *Leblanc* (1975) for isolated frog skin. The decline in I_{Na}^m conforms to a single exponential function of time after exposure to Na and is described by the relation:

$$(I_{Na}^m)_t = 3 \exp^{-6.9t} + 2 \ (\mu Eq/cm^2hr).$$

Extrapolation of this curve to zero-time yields an amiloride-sensitive Na entry rate of 5 $\mu Eq/cm^2hr$. That is, the initial rate of Na entry into Na-depleted tissues is in excellent agreement with the maximal rate of the basolateral Na pump mechanism in the presence of 140 mM Na (*Frizzell* and *Turnheim*, 1978; *Turnheim*, *Frizzell*, and *Schultz*, 1978). In addition, the amiloride-sensitive component of G_t ($_aG_{Na}$) obtained from these studies follows a similar time course (data not shown) and decreases from a maximal value at zero-time of 1.7 mmhos/cm² to a value of 0.7 mmhos/cm² in the steady-state.

As previously discussed (*Schultz, Frizzell,* and *Nellans,* 1977), electrophysiologic considerations indicate that this must represent a decrease in the conductance of the mucosal membrane to Na. Thus, the maximal values of I_{Na}^m and $_aG_{Na}$ observed in Na-depleted tissues are in good agreement with those associated with maximal rates of Na extrusion from cell to serosal solution across the basolateral membranes (e.g., spontaneous or induced by the presence of stimulatory anions). However, these findings suggest that the permeability of the entry step to Na is progressively reduced from its maximal value as repletion of the intracellular Na content occurs.

A possible explanation for the results given in Figure 1 emerges from a comparison of the amount of Na which enters the colonic mucosa

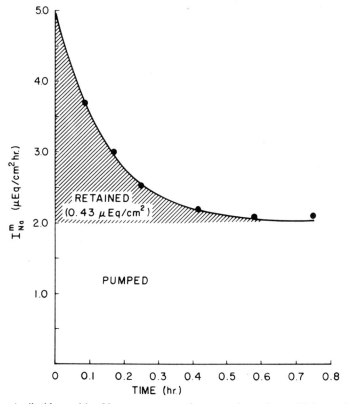

Fig. 1.   Amiloride-sensitive Na current across the mucosal membrane (I_{Na}^m) as a function of time following exposure of Na-depleted tissues to 140 mM Na. The rationale for dividing the total I_{Na}^m into Na retained by the tissue and Na pumped from mucosa-to-serosa is detailed in the text.

during the transient in I_{Na}^m and the exchangeable Na content of this tissue (*Frizzell*, unpublished observations). When the tissues are exposed to a Na-free mucosal solution for 30–45 min, cell Na content declines from a control level of 0.55 μEq/cm^2 to a value of 0.15 μEq/cm^2. Thus, approximately 0.40 μEq/cm^2 of the total intracellular Na appears to be accessible by Na in the mucosal solution. This value is in excellent agreement with the area under the transient overshoot of I_{Na}^m shown in Figure 1 (0.43 μEq/cm^2) during the period from zero-time, representing the time of exposure of Na-depleted cells to 140 mM Na in the mucosal solution, to 0.6 hr, representing the time at which steady-state values of I_{Na}^m (equal to J_{net}^{Na}) are achieved. Thus, the Na which enters the cells during the transient of I_{Na}^m appears to have two fates: that which comprises the transient (cross-hatched portion in Fig. 1) is sufficient to replete the normal cellular Na content accessible from the mucosal solution and is therefore retained within the tissue; and the remainder of the Na which enters the cells from zero-time would permit transepithelial Na transport at the rate of 2 μEq/cm^{2}hr (the steady-state rate) from zero-time. According to this analysis, transcellular Na transport proceeds at, or close to, the steady-state level from the outset. Thus, the negative feedback effect of cell Na on its entry across the mucosal membrane arises

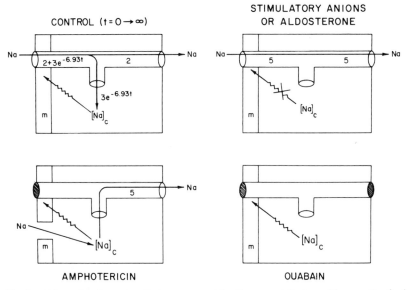

Fig. 2.   Schematic of a system that can account for the present findings. The negative feedback effect of [Na]$_c$ on the Na permeability of the entry step is represented by the jagged arrow. Blockage of the entry or exit steps of active Na transport pathway is depicted by cross-hatching.

from a cellular compartment that is not directly involved in trans-epithelial Na transport under normal conditions. In other words, the decline in I^m_{Na} shown in Figure 1 appears to be closely related to repletion of the intracellular Na content.

Figure 2 illustrates a system that is consistent with this interpretation. The pathway responsible for active, transcellular Na transport is shown to run in parallel with the major cellular Na compartment with which it communicates. The Na content of the active transport pathway is considered to be very small so that it fills rapidly following exposure of Na-depleted cells to Na, and steady-state rates of active transcellular Na transport are quickly achieved. This conclusion is consistent with that of *Cereijido, et al.* (1974) for isolated frog skin. A second Na compartment, comprising the bulk of cell Na, appears to be responsible for the negative feedback effect on amiloride-sensitive Na entry. Thus, at zero-time, when cell Na is low, entry is maximal; however, as Na enters, the Na content of cellular compartment, $[Na]_c$, is slowly restored, and as this occurs, the permeability of the entry step is reduced until a steady-state is achieved, where $I^m_{Na} = J^{Na}_{net}$.[2]

It should be stressed that these conclusions would not be compromised even if our estimates of the area under the overshoot of I^m_{Na} (Fig. 1) or the amount of cell Na derived from the mucosal solution were in error by as much as 30%, which seems very unlikely. Thus, transcellular Na transport achieves steady-state levels long before $[Na]_c$ is repleted, and the decrease in I^m_{Na} and the conductance of the amiloride-sensitive entry step appear to be related to repletion of $[Na]_c$ and not to the Na content of the active Na transport pool. This negative feedback effect would serve to regulate $[Na]_c$ and "protect" it when pump activity becomes rate-limiting.

Also shown in Figure 2 are possible explanations for the effects of agents which alter the rate of transepithelial Na transport and the conductance of the Na entry step in rabbit colon. Stimulatory anions and aldosterone may give rise to maximal rates of Na absorption by interrupting the negative feedback effect of $[Na]_c$ in some as yet unknown manner. Amphotericin may enhance J^{Na}_{net} by increasing $[Na]_c$, which at the same time would block the normal, amiloride-sensitive entry process

---

[2] The amiloride-sensitive component of the transepithelial current (I_{sc}) can clearly be identified with the net flow of Na across the mucosal membrane (I^m_{Na}), at all points in time. However, during the transient in I_{sc} which follows exposure of Na-depleted tissues to 140 mM Na, movements of Na as well as other ions may contribute to the current across the basolateral membranes. Studies of cell composition (*Frizzell*, unpublished observations) indicate that exposure of tissues to Na-free mucosal solutions leads to decreased NaCl (and H_2O) content with no change in K content. Thus, a portion of the current across the basolateral membrane during the transient is probably due to entry of Cl into the cells from the serosal solution.

(Table 1). Finally, ouabain, by blocking exit of Na from the active transport pathway, would lead to an increase in $[Na]_c$ and, as with amphotericin, result in a blockage of entry. These conclusions appear to provide a mechanistic basis for the findings that metabolic inhibitors or exposure to low temperatures decrease the rate of Na entry across the outer barrier or mucosal membranes of Na-transporting epithelia, so that an active Na entry process (*Biber*, 1971; *Moreno et al.*, 1973) need not be invoked to account for these observations. A decrease in mucosal membrane Na permeability secondary to an increase in cell Na content can readily account for these findings.

SUMMARY

The effects of a number of agents or conditions which modify trans-epithelial Na transport by rabbit colon are summarized in Figure 3. The conductance of the amiloride-sensitive, active Na transport pathway, $_aG_{Na}$, and the net flow of Na across the mucosal membrane, I_{Na}^m (which under steady-state conditions equals J_{net}^{Na}) are illustrated. Several of these observations can be explained on the basis of a negative feedback effect of cell Na on the Na conductance of the mucosal cell membrane, which will be reflected by changes in $_aG_{Na}$. Thus, upon exposure of Na-depleted cells to 140 mM Na-Ringer's, $_aG_{Na}$ and I_{Na}^m are maximal. As cell Na concentrations rise with Na repletion, $_aG_{Na}$ and I_{Na}^m decrease until steady-state values are reached. The steady-state value of $_aG_{Na}$ is considered to depend upon the size of the intracellular Na pool ($[Na]_c$). If $[Na]_c$ is elevated, as a consequence of addition of ouabain or amphotericin, $_aG_{Na}$ is abolished. In the case of ouabain, J_{net}^{Na} is also abolished since exit is blocked; but with amphotericin, a maximal rate of Na absorption is observed since amiloride-sensitive Na entry is no longer the rate-limiting step in transepithelial Na transport. The stimulatory anions or aldosterone elicit the maximal I_{Na}^m in the presence of 140 mM Na; as discussed above, these agents may interfere with the normal feedback effect of $[Na]_c$. Although this possibility is speculative, phenomenologically the system behaves as if $[Na]_c \cong 0$. Clearly, amiloride results in a direct blockage of the Na entry step which abolishes $_aG_{Na}$ and reduces I_{Na}^m to zero.

According to the classical series-membrane model of transepithelial Na transport (*Koefoed-Johnsen* and *Ussing*, 1958), variations in J_{net} are normally considered to involve changes in either the rate of Na entry into the transporting cells or the activity of the mechanism responsible for Na extrusion from the cells across the basolateral membranes. In terms of alterations in the Na permeability of the mucosal membrane, the nega-

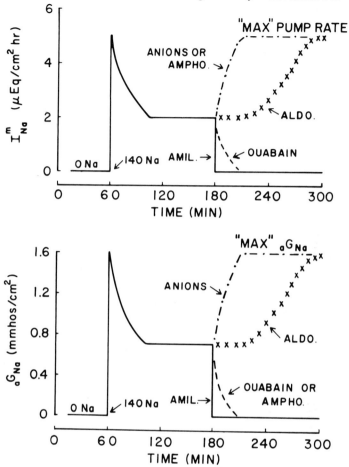

Fig. 3. Summary of effects of various agents or conditions altering the rate of transepithelial Na transport. Changes in I_{Na}^m and $_aG_{Na}$ are depicted as arbitrary functions of time, but the time course of each effect is relatively accurate.

tive feedback effect of $[Na]_c$ represents a potential site of interaction for agents that stimulate or inhibit transepithelial Na transport.

REFERENCES

Biber, T.U.L. 1971. Effect of changes in transepithelial transport on the uptake of sodium across the outer surface of the frog skin. J Gen Physiol 53:131–144

Cereijido, M., C.A. Rabito, E. Rodriguez Boulan and C.A. Rotunno 1974. The sodium-transporting compartment of the epithelium of frog skin. J Physiol (London) 237:555–571

Cuthbert, A.W. and W.K. Shum 1971. Does intracellular sodium modify membrane permeability to sodium ions? Nature (London) 266:468–469

Erlij, D. and M.W. Smith 1973. Sodium uptake by frog skin and its modification by inhibitors of transepithelial sodium transport. J Physiol (London) 228:221–239

Essig, A. and A. Leaf. 1963. The role of potassium in active transport of sodium by the toad bladder. J Gen Physiol 46:505–515

Finn, A.L. 1975. Action of ouabain on sodium transport in toad urinary bladder. Evidence for two pathways for sodium entry. J Gen Physiol 65:503–514

Frizzell, R.A., M.J. Koch and S.G. Schultz 1976. Ion transport by rabbit colon. I. Active and passive components. J Membrane Biol 27:297–316

Frizzell, R.A. and S.G. Schultz. 1978. Effect of aldosterone on ion transport by rabbit colon in vitro. J Membrane Biol 39:1–26

Frizzell, R.A. and K. Turnheim. 1978. Ion transport by rabbit colon: II. Unidirectional sodium influx and the effects of amphotericin B and amiloride. J Membrane Biol 40:193–211

Helman, S.I. and W. Nagel. 1977. Microelectrode studies of frog skin. Effects of ouabain. Fed Proc 36:632

Koefoed-Johnsen, V. and H.H. Ussing. 1958. The nature of the frog skin potential. Acta Physiol Scand 42:298–308

Larsen, E.H. 1973. Effect of amiloride, cyanide and ouabain on the active transport pathway in toad skin. In Transport Mechanisms in Epithelia, eds. H.H. Ussing and N.A. Thorn, pp. 131–143. Copenhagen: Munksgaard

Lewis, S.A., D.C. Eaton and J.M. Diamond. 1976. The mechanism of Na transport by rabbit urinary bladder. J Membrane Biol 28:41–70

MacRobbie, E.A.C. and H.H.Ussing. 1961. Osmotic behavior of the epithelial cells of frog skin. Acta Physiol Scand 53:348–365

Morel, F. and G. Leblanc. 1975. Transient current changes and Na compartmentalization in frog skin epithelium. Pfluger's Arch 358:135–157

Moreno, J.H., I.L. Reisin, E. Rodriguez Boulan, C.A. Rotunno and M. Cereijido. 1973. Barriers to sodium movement across frog skin epithelium. J Membrane Biol 11:99–115

Phillips, S.F. and P.F. Schmalz. 1970. Bicarbonate secretion by the rat colon. Effect of intraluminal chloride and acetazolamide. Proc Soc Exp Biol Med 135:116–122

Rick, R., A. Dörge and W. Nagel. 1975. Influx and efflux of sodium at the outer surface of frog skin. J Membrane Biol 22:183–196

Robinson, B.A. and A.D.C. Macknight. 1976. Relationships between serosal medium potassium concentration and sodium transport in toad urinary bladder. II. Effects of different medium potassium concentrations on epithelial cell composition. J Membrane Biol 26:239–268

Schultz, S.G., R.A. Frizzell and H.N. Nellans 1977. Active sodium transport and the electrophysiology of rabbit colon. J Membrane Biol 33:351–384

Turnheim, K., R.A. Frizzell and S.G. Schultz 1977. Effect of anions on amiloride-sensitive, active sodium transport across rabbit colon, in vitro. Evidence for "trans-inhibition" of the sodium entry mechanism. J Membrane Biol 37:63–84

Turnheim, K., R.A. Frizzell and S.G. Schultz. 1978. Interaction between cell sodium and the amiloride-sensitive sodium entry step in rabbit colon. J Membrane Biol, 39:233–256

© 1979 Urban & Schwarzenberg, Inc. Baltimore-Munich
Amiloride and Epithelial Sodium Transport
Edited by A.W. Cuthbert, G.M. Fanelli, Jr. and A. Scriabine

Studies of the Na⁺ Channel in Cultured Dog Kidney Epithelial Cells Utilizing Amiloride

Mary Taub

Department of Biology
The University of California, San Diego
La Jolla, California 92093

INTRODUCTION

The dog kidney epithelial cell line MDCK (Madin Darby Canine Kidney) is a novel model system for examining the mechanisms by which solutes are transported across kidney epithelia. That MDCK cells have differentiated properties of kidney cells was first suggested by *Leighton et al.* (1970) who observed the occurrence of hemicysts, or blisters, in MDCK cell cultures. The hemicysts are regions on a MDCK monolayer where the cells are slightly elevated from the Petri dish surface. Hemicyst formation has been attributed to the vectorial transport of salt and water from the mucosal surface of the cells (facing the medium) to the serosal surface (facing the dish). These transepithelial transport processes have been shown to occur in MDCK cells by *Misfeldt, Hamamoto,* and *Pitelka* (1976) utilizing a Ussing chamber. MDCK cells also retain hormone responses unique to distal tubule cells (*Rindler, Chuman,* and *Saier,* in preparation), and thus provide the opportunity to examine the mechanisms by which hormones regulate salt and water flux. Toward these ends, *Taub* (1978) and *Rindler, Taub,* and *Saier* (in preparation) have examined the mechanism of Na⁺ transport by the Na⁺ channel in MDCK cells both kinetically and genetically (*Taub, Rindler,* and *Saier,* 1977). Amiloride has been utilized in these studies as a selective reagent for obtaining mutants with an altered Na⁺ channel.

MATERIALS AND METHODS

Cell Maintenance and Cell Growth Studies

MDCK cells and amiloride-resistant variants of MDCK were maintained as monolayer cultures in Dulbecco's Modified Eagle's Medium

(DME) containing 10% fetal calf serum. To determine the effect of amiloride on cell growth, cells were distributed at 5×10^4 cells/dish into 60 mm Petri dishes containing 4 ml DME and amiloride; after an appropriate incubation period at 37°C in a 5% CO_2, 95% air incubator, the cell number was determined using a Coulter counter.

Transport Studies

The incorporation of labeled substrate into the intracellular compartment was studied using confluent monolayer cultures of cells in 35 mm tissue culture dishes. Uptake of labeled solute ($^{22}Na^+$, $^{86}Rb^+$, ^{14}C-amiloride, $^{45}Ca^{++}$) occurred at 24°C using either 1 mM Tris-HCl buffer or phosphate buffered saline (PBS), pH 7.3, made isotonic to physiological saline with sucrose as a Na^+ replacement. Cells were routinely washed using 110 mM Tris buffer, the intracellular label was extracted into deionized water for at least 1 hr, and label was counted in Triton-based PPO/POPOP. Uptake determinations were made in duplicate (or in triplicate when determining Michaelis-Menton constants), and corrected for zero-time uptake (label not removed by the washing procedure). Prior to studying Na^+ influx through the channel, MDCK cells were preincubated for at least 1 hr in DME containing 10^{-5} M ouabain at 37°C, conditions which have been shown to permit maximal inhibition of Na^+/K^+ ATPase activity. To determine Michaelis-Menton constants, the initial rate of Na^+ uptake was determined using a 5-min time interval, and was corrected for diffusion as described.

CO_2 Evolution

The evolution of CO_2 from 2-^{14}C-pyruvate was determined using cell monolayers maintained in 30 mm Ehrlenmeyer flasks. Prior to adding labeled pyruvate and amiloride, monolayers were equilibrated at 37°C for 1 hr in a 5% CO_2, 95% air incubator, in Minimal Essential Medium (MEM) containing 10% dialyzed fetal calf serum. Then labeled pyruvate (3.8×10^{-5} M, 6.6 mCi/μM) was added to the flasks; sealed flasks were incubated at 37°C. After the incubation period, labeled material in each flask was captured in a well containing 0.4 ml 8 M NaOH, after acidifying the medium (MEM) with TCA. The labeled CO_2 was counted in Triton-Toluene scintillation fluid. Determinations were in duplicate and corrected for zero-time CO_2 evolution.

Chemicals

Both amiloride and ^{14}C-amiloride were gifts from Merck & Co., Inc., Rahway, N.J. Other radiochemicals ($^{22}Na^+$, $^{86}Rb^+$, $^{45}Ca^{++}$ 2-^{14}C-pyruvate) were obtained from New England Nuclear.

RESULTS

Kinetics of Na$^+$ Transport in MDCK Cells

Na$^+$ transport via the Na$^+$ channel in MDCK cells is a saturable process (Fig. 1) (*Taub, Rindler*, and *Saier*, 1977) subject to exchange diffusion of two types: a) Na$^+$/Na$^+$ exchange, and b) Na$^+$/proton antiport. The latter process has been observed in cells located in the distal portion of the kidney nephron (see *Koushanpour*, 1976). Although hormonal regulation of Na$^+$ transport has not been demonstrated in MDCK cells, calcium has been implicated as an important regulatory molecule for Na$^+$ uptake via the channel (*Taub et al.*, 1977). While extracellular calcium is inhibitory to Na$^+$ influx, intracellular calcium stimulates the influx process, a phenomenon which may result from allosteric effects of calcium on the Na$^+$ channel. The diuretic drug, amiloride, inhibits Na$^+$ influx in MDCK cells, as would be expected of epithelial cells of kidney origin. The inhibition of Na$^+$ uptake caused by extracellular amiloride follows the kinetics of a partial or mixed inhibition system as indicated by the nonlinear Dixon plot (Fig. 2). A nonlinear Dixon plot also is observed when using calcium as a Na$^+$ transport inhibitor, although to obtain 50% inhibition of 1.1 mM Na$^+$ influx 1.8×10^{-3} M calcium is necessary, as compared

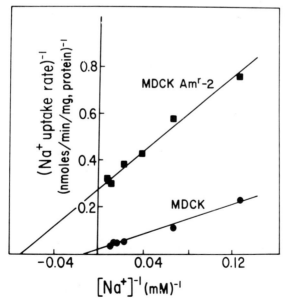

Fig. 1. Lineweaver-Burk plot of Na$^+$ uptake. The initial rate of Na$^+$ uptake was determined between 1.1 and 110 mM NaCl using both MDCK and Am^{r}2, as described in Materials and Methods. The uptake was corrected for diffusion and plotted on a double reciprocal plot.

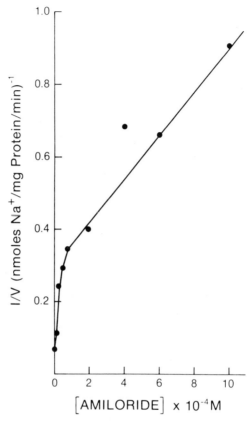

Fig. 2.   Dixon plot of amiloride inhibition of Na$^+$ influx. The inhibitory effect of amiloride on 1.1 mM ^{22}Na$^+$ uptake was determined using a 5-min time interval. Uptake determinations were in duplicate.

to 1.5×10^{-5} M amiloride (unpublished observation). In the distal tubule of rat kidney 2×10^{-6} M amiloride causes 50% inhibition of Na$^+$ absorption (*Meng*, 1975), while much higher concentrations (1000-fold) were required to inhibit uptake in the proximal tubule.

Amiloride-resistant Mutants

The observation that amiloride is inhibitory to Na$^+$ transport indicated that the drug could be used as a selective reagent for isolating mutants with alterations in the Na$^+$ channel from MDCK cell cultures. In a similar manner, ouabain has been used as a selective reagent to obtain mutants with an altered Na$^+$/K$^+$ ATPase from cultured Chinese hamster ovary cells (*Baker, et al.*, 1974).

Amiloride at 3×10^{-4} M is cytotoxic to MDCK cells, and over a dozen independent clones of cells resistant to killing by 3×10^{-4} M amiloride have been isolated from mutagenized MDCK cell cultures (*Taub*, unpublished observation). All six of the resistant clones tested were partially resistant to the growth inhibition caused by amiloride at 2.5 to 7.5 $\times$ 10^{-4} M. The amiloride-resistant phenotype is stable over a 6-month period of growth in nonselective medium; in addition, the frequency of resistant clones in MDCK cell cultures is enhanced by mutagen treatment from 2 $\times$ 10^{-5} to 6 $\times$ 10^{-4} M in cultures treated with 2 μg/ml nitrosoguanidine. These observations are consistent with the hypothesis that the varient clones arose as a result of mutational events rather than by epigenetic changes.

All of the resistant clones studied were distinguished from MDCK cells microscopically. While hemicysts were observed in confluent monolayers of MDCK cells, no such hemicysts were observed in confluent cultures of amiloride-resistant clones Am^{r}2, Am^{r}4, and Am^{r}22. This observation suggested that the amiloride-resistant cells were defective in transepithelial transport of salt or water, processes which have been proposed to play an important role in hemicyst formation (*Abaza*, *Leighton*, and *Schultz*, 1974).

Thus, Na$^+$ transport was examined in MDCK and an amiloride-resistant clone, Am^{r}2. Figure 3 illustrates the time course of Na$^+$ influx in amiloride-resistant clone Am^{r}2 and MDCK in the presence or absence of ouabain. Incubation with ouabain increases the Na$^+$ entry rate to a greater extent in MDCK than in Am^{r}2. The reduced Na$^+$ uptake rate in Am^{r}2 is not easily explained by an alteration in the Na$^+$/K$^+$ ATPase as in both MDCK and Am^{r}2 the rate of ouabain-sensitive Rb$^+$ influx and the sensitivity of Rb$^+$ influx to inhibition by ouabain do not differ significantly. Thus, reduced Na$^+$ transport is explainable by an alteration in the activity of the Na$^+$ channel in Am^{r}2. Lineweaver-Burke plots of Na$^+$ uptake in MDCK and Am^{r}2 are linear (Fig. 1), and in Am^{r}2 both the Km and Vm for Na$^+$ uptake were altered. While in MDCK the Km and Vm for Na$^+$ uptake were 75 mM and 40 nmoles Na$^+$/min/mg protein, respectively, in Am^{r}2 the Km and Vm were 14 mM and 3.7 nmoles/min/mg protein, respectively. These results indicate that a structural gene mutation affecting the Na$^+$ channel may have occurred in Am^{r}2.

Transport of Other Molecules by Am^{r}2

Cation inhibition studies indicate that Na$^+$, Li$^+$, K$^+$, Rb$^+$ and guanidine are competitive inhibitors of Na$^+$ uptake (*Rindler*, *Taub*, and *Saier*, in preparation), with similar capacities to inhibit Na$^+$ influx via the Na$^+$ channel (Table 1). As these studies indicate that in MDCK cells the Na$^+$ channel is actually a general cation transport system, the possibility was considered that Am^{r}2 transports other cations at reduced rates. The initial rates of ouabain-insensitive Rb$^+$ influx and Ca^{++} influx were

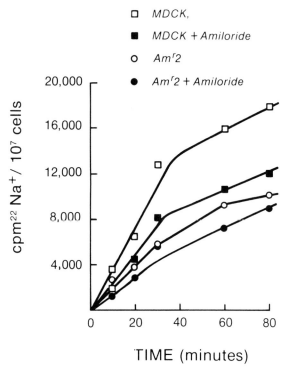

Fig. 3. Time course of Na⁺ uptake in DME in MDCK and Amʳ2. Na⁺ uptake in MDCK and Amʳ2 was examined in DME containing 110 mm Na plus ^{22}Na⁺ over an 80-min period. Uptake proceeded either in the presence or absence of 10^{-5} M ouabain at 37°C in a 5% CO_2, 95% air incubator. One hour prior to the uptake period, the medium was changed either to DME or DME + 10^{-5} M ouabain in the presence or absence of 10^{-2} M amiloride. Uptake determinations, made in duplicate, were standardized with respect to cell number.

examined and were observed to be lower in Amʳ2 than in MDCK. However, the rates of ouabain-sensitive Rb⁺ influx and αAIBA influx do not differ in MDCK and Amʳ2, indicating that a generalized change in membrane transport has not occurred in MDCK cells.

Mechanism of Resistance to Killing by Amiloride

Amiloride may kill MDCK cells by preventing Na⁺ transport through the Na⁺ channel; alternatively, the drug may kill the cells by its effects intracellularly. In MDCK cells 10^{-2} M amiloride inhibited both Na⁺ and Ca⁺⁺ transport by 30% in DME; less inhibition of uptake was observed in Amʳ2. However, at lower amiloride concentrations (10^{-3} M) no significant inhibition of either Na⁺ or Ca⁺⁺ influx was observed. As 10^{-3} M is slightly higher than the amiloride concentration used for isolating resistant clones, it seemed unlikely that amiloride killed cells by its inhibitory effects on cation transport. Thus, the hypothesis was investigated that amiloride killed MDCK cells by inhibiting an intracellular function. Initial observations indicated that killing by amiloride could be prevented by routinely replacing the growth medium with fresh medium (DME containing amiloride).

As further studies suggested that the cytotoxic effects of amiloride depended upon the utilization of nutrients from the medium rather than the accumulation of a toxic byproduct of amiloride, the ability of several nutrients to relieve killing by the drug was studied. After 3 days of incubation with amiloride at 7.5×10^{-4} M, nutrients were added to the culture medium at concentrations used in DME. While the addition of glucose, the essential amino acids or vitamins had no significant effect on cell number, the addition of fresh serum or pyruvate at 5 mM not only prevented cell death but partially relieved the growth inhibition caused by the drug. These observations are explainable if cell death is due to inhibitory effects of amiloride on the TCA cycle (*Losert et al.*, 1969).

That amiloride does have a mitochondrial site of action was further indicated by CO_2 evolution studies (Fig. 4). In amiloride-resistant clone Am^{r}2 amiloride was less inhibitory to CO_2 evolution from pyruvate than in MDCK cells. These results indicate that amiloride kills MDCK cells by inhibiting mitochondrial function, and that in Am^{r}2 cell death does not occur, as mitochondrial function is no longer impaired. Assuming cell death occurs as a consequence of amiloride's mitochondrial effects,

Table 1.   Cation Competition Study*

	Amiloride Uptake	Total Rb$^+$ Uptake	% Standard Influx Ouabain-Insensitive Rb$^+$ Uptake	Na$^+$ Uptake
Std. (none)	100 ± 6	100 ± 7	100 ± 3	100 ± 15
LiCl	66 ± 3	99 ± 1	46 ± 3	40 ± 2
NaCl	62 ± 6	122 ± 3	42 ± 3	38 ± 12
Guanidine HCl	53 ± 7	93 ± 2	28 ± 6	37 ± 20
KCl	64 ± 6	59 ± 2	26 ± 2	35 ± 6
Amiloride	15 ± 2			
Ouabain		34 ± 1	100 ± 3	

* The inhibitory effect of cations on the initial rate of ^{86}Rb$^+$, ^{14}C-Amiloride and ^{22}Na$^+$ uptake was studied using labeled Rb$^+$, amiloride and Na$^+$ at 1 mM, 0.035 mM and 1.1 mM, respectively. Unlabeled competing cations were present at 11 mM to inhibit amiloride and Rb$^+$ influx, and at 55 mM to inhibit Na$^+$ influx. Competing cations were added simultaneously with the reaction mixture containing labeled cation. Uptake proceeded over a 4-min period in 1 mM Tris, 6% sucrose buffer. One hour prior to examining Rb$^+$ influx, the medium was changed to DME (to study total influx), or to DME $+ 10^{-5}$ M ouabain (to study ouabain-insensitive Rb$^+$ influx). Uptake determinations were made in triplicate.

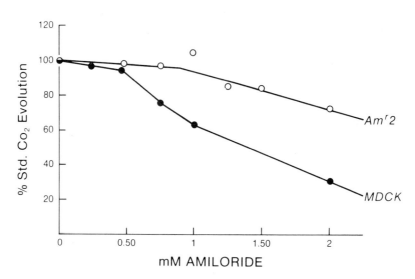

Fig. 4.   Effect of amiloride on CO_2 evolution from pyruvate. CO_2 evolution from 2-^{14}C-pyruvate was determined in confluent monolayers of MDCK and Am^{r}2 incubated in the presence or absence of amiloride (0-2 $\times$ 10^{-3} M) for a 10-hr time interval, as described in Materials and Methods.

the mechanism by which an alteration affecting the Na$^+$ channel could confer resistance to killing was studied. [14C]-labeled amiloride uptake into mutant and wild-type MDCK cells was examined (Fig. 5). Both the initial rate of uptake and the steady-state level of accumulation were lower in Am^{r}2 than in MDCK. This defect could have resulted from a mutation affecting the entry of amiloride into MDCK by a transport system or free diffusion. However, cation competition studies indicated that amiloride accumulation was inhibited by guanidine, Na$^+$ and Ca^{++}, cations which inhibit ouabain-insensitive Na$^+$ influx through the Na$^+$ channel; ouabain had only a minor effect on the accumulation process (Table 1). These results suggest that amiloride enters MDCK via the Na$^+$ channel, and they provide supporting evidence for the hypothesis that the mutational alteration in Am^{r}2 decreases the extent of amiloride accumulation, thereby preventing cell death.

DISCUSSION

Na$^+$ transport by the Na$^+$ channel in MDCK cell is a saturable process subject to accelerative exchange diffusion with intracellular Na$^+$, or protons, and regulation by both intracellular and extracellular calcium. Na$^+$ transport in MDCK cells is sensitive to inhibition by amiloride. A Dixon plot of the amiloride inhibition of Na$^+$ transport is nonlinear, as has also been observed for inhibition by extracellular calcium. Utilizing the drug as a selective reagent, "mutant" clones which are partially resistant to growth inhibition by amiloride have been isolated from MDCK cell cultures. The amiloride-resistant clones are defective not only in hemicyst formation but also in the rate of Na^+ influx by the Na^+ channel. One resistant clone, Am^r2, has an alteration in the Km and Vm for Na^+ uptake by the channel, which suggests (but does not necessarily indicate) that a structural gene mutation has occurred in Am^r2. Ouabain-insensitive Rb^+ influx and calcium influx occur at reduced rates in Am^r2, which may be explained if these cations are transported by the Na^+ channel. However, the possibility cannot be excluded that the alteration in the activity of the Na^+ channel is actually due to a generalized membrane change.

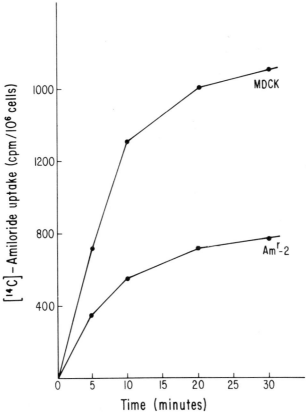

Fig. 5.   Time course of amiloride uptake in MDCK and Am^r2. The uptake of 3.5×10^{-5} M ^{14}C-amiloride was examined over a 25-min period in Tris buffer. Uptake determinations were made in duplicate every 5 min during the uptake period.

Alternatively, amiloride resistance may be conferred as a result of a mitochondrial mutation, which indirectly affects uptake by the Na^+ channel. In considering this possibility, we have presented evidence indicating that amiloride does affect mitochondrial function. Not only is the evolution of CO_2 from pyruvate inhibited upon incubation with the drug, but the addition of excess pyruvate to the medium prevents the cytotoxic effects of amiloride. In addition, fluorescent microscope studies indicate that amiloride (a highly fluorescent compound) is concentrated in the mitochondria. In these studies a correlation was made between the fluorescent organelles observed in MDCK cells incubated with amiloride, and organelles stained using fluorescene-conjugated antibody to cytochrome oxidase, a mitochondrial marker (*Taub* and *Louvard*, unpublished observations). Thus, conceivably the mitochondrion is the site at which amiloride acts, so as to cause MDCK cell death. Consistent with this hypothesis is the observation that amiloride treatment causes less inhibition of CO_2 evolution from pyruvate in amiloride-resistant clone Am^r2 than in MDCK cells. The latter observation also could be interpreted as indicating that the primary defect in Am^r2 is in the mitochondria, rather than in the cell membrane. Presumably, a mitochondrial change could indirectly affect the activity of the Na^+ channel, a hypothesis which has been proposed previously regarding a possible mechanism of action of aldosterone (*Losert et al.*, 1969).

The evidence which has been presented, however, is consistent with the hypothesis that an alteration in the Na^+ channel confers resistance to killing by amiloride in clone Am^r2. According to this hypothesis, amiloride enters the cells at a reduced rate, so that the intracellular drug concentration is reduced below the level necessary to inhibit mitochondrial function. Further studies will be concerned with determining the location of the primary defects in amiloride-resistant clone Am^r2, as well as the other resistant clones studied.

REFERENCES

Abaza, N.A., Leighton, J., and Schultz, S.G. 1974. Effects of ouabain on the function and structure of a cell line (MDCK) derived from canine kidney. I. Light microscopic observations of monolayer growth. In Vitro 10:172–183

Baker, R.M., Brunette, O.M., Mankovitz, R., Thompson, L.H., Whitmore, G.F., Siminovitch, L., and Till, J.E. 1974. Ouabain-resistant mutants of mouse and hamster cells in culture. Cell 1:9–21

Koushanpour, E. 1976. *Renal Physiology, Principles and Functions*. Philadelphia: Saunders, p. 336

Leighton, J.L., Estes, W., Musukhani, S., and Brada, Z. 1970. A cell line derived from normal dog kidney (MDCK) exhibiting properties of papillary adenocarcinoma of renal tubular epithelium. Cancer 26:1022–1028

Losert, W., Sitt, R., Senft, G., Bergmann, K.V., and Zesch, A. 1969. Biochemical Studies on Mechanisms of Action of Compounds Influencing Tubular Na$^+$ Transport: Aldosterone, Amiloride and Triamterene. In *Progress in Nephrology*, eds. G. Peters and F. Roch-Ramel, p. 267–274, Berlin: Springer-Verlag

Meng, K. 1974. Comparison of local effects of amiloride hydrochloride on the isotonic fluid absorption in the distal and proximal convoluted tubule. Pflügers Arch 357:91–99

Misfeldt, D.S., Hamamoto, S.T., and Pitelka, D.R. 1976. Transepithelial transport in cell culture. Proc Nat Acad Sci USA 73:1212–1216

Rindler, M.J., Chuman, L., and Saier, M.H., Jr. 1979. Isolation of amiloride-resistant clones from dog kidney epithelial cells. J Cell Biol, in press

Rindler, M.J., Taub, M., and Saier, M.H., Jr. in preparation

Taub, M. 1978. Somatic cell genetics, 4:609–616

Taub, M., Rindler, M.J., and Saier, M.H., Jr. 1977. ^{22}Na$^+$ Transport in an established kidney epithelial cell line (MDCK). J Cell Biol 75:368a

Na⁺ Transport and Swelling of the Mammalian Blastocyst: Effect of Amiloride

John D. Biggers* and R. Douglas Powers**

** Department of Physiology and Laboratory of Human
Reproduction and Reproductive Biology
Harvard Medical School
Boston, Massachusetts 02115
** Department of Biology
Boston College
Chestnut Hill, Massachusetts 02167*

INTRODUCTION

During the first few days of development the mammalian embryo divides mitotically to form a ball of cells called the morula. This ball of cells then accumulates fluid internally to give rise to the blastocyst. Scanning electron micrographs of this developmental sequence in the mouse are shown in Figure 1. At first the individual cells are very discrete and are held together loosely. Eventually a stage of development is reached where the individual cells become intimately associated, and their boundaries can no longer be easily recognized. This sudden loss of cell identity is sufficiently pronounced that classical embryologists coined the term "compaction" to denote the event (*Lewis* and *Gregory*, 1929). It is known now that compaction is associated with the formation of tight junctions between the outer trophoblast cells of the morula and that this process results in the formation of the first tissue in the new multicellular organism (*Schlafke* and *Enders*, 1967; *Calarco* and *Brown*, 1969; *Ducibella et al.*, 1975; *Hastings* and *Enders*, 1975; *Izquierdo*, *Fernandez*, and *Lopez*, 1976). The tissue, called the trophectoderm, is a simple squamous epithelium that provides the integument of the late preimplantation embryo.

The preparation of this paper was supported in part by grants from the Rockefeller Foundation, RF 65040 and RF 77045, and the National Institute of Child Health and Human Development, HD-06916-04.

167

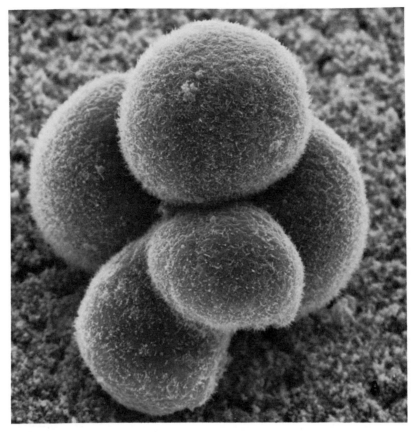

Fig. 1A.   Four-cell mouse embryo with one dividing blastomere. From *Ducibella et al.*, J
Cell Biol 74:153–167, 1977.

FUNCTIONAL CONSEQUENCES OF COMPACTION

The development of a functional integument in the preimplantation
embryo provides the machinery for establishing an extracellular fluid.
This fluid has at least two functions which are related to separate compartments. The smaller compartment provides the milieu intérieur for the
cells of the inner cell mass, and may govern their pattern of differentiation (*Tarkowski* and *Wroblewska*, 1967; *Hillman, Sherman,* and
Graham, 1972). The larger compartment is the blastocoele fluid, whose
accumulation causes swelling of the blastocyst that may be necessary for
the attachment reaction (*Nilsson*, 1967). The remainder of this paper will
be concerned only with the blastocoele fluid, since nothing is known
about the composition of the microenvironment of the cells of the inner
cell mass.

Figure 2 illustrates the effects of compaction by comparing theoretical models for the pre- and post-compacted embryos. The major change is the establishment of vectorial transport systems that move substances across the trophectoderm. These systems, as in all other epithelia, involve both transcellular and paracellular routes. Although the systems are open, they have major constraints since all substances must pass through compartment 1.

Compartment 5 has the important developmental property that it increases in size. The factors that affect this process control the rate of growth of the blastocyst and its ultimate dimensions. The blastocysts of all mammals expand, but there is tremendous variation between species in the extent of the expansion (*Biggers*, 1972). At one extreme is the minimally expanding type, e.g., the mouse, which increases in volume only 5- to 7-fold; at the other extreme is the maximally expanding type, e.g., the rabbit, which increases in volume by several orders of mag-

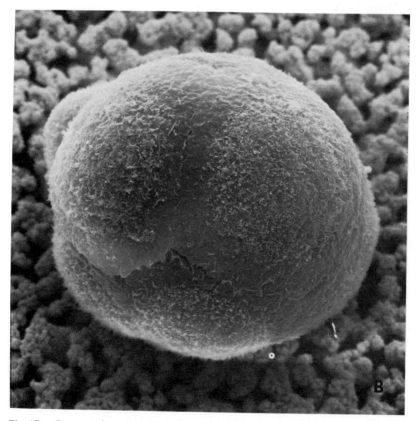

Fig. 1B.   Compacted mouse embryo. From *Ducibella et al.*, J Cell Biol 74:153–167, 1977.

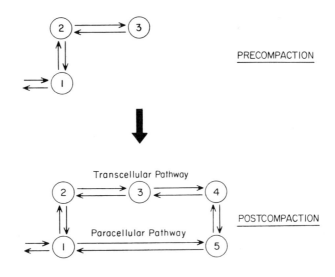

THEORETICAL MODELS OF
PRE- AND POST- COMPACTED EMBRYOS

PRECOMPACTION

Transcellular Pathway

POSTCOMPACTION

Paracellular Pathway

I - UTERINE FLUID
2 - OUTER MEMBRANE COMPARTMENT (abcoelic compartment)
3 - INTRACELLULAR COMPARTMENT
4 - INNER MEMBRANE COMPARTMENT (juxtacoelic compartment)
5 - BLASTOCOELE FLUID

Fig. 2.   Theoretical models showing the effect of compaction in the transport of substances in the early mammalian embryo.

nitude. The large changes in the rabbit blastocyst make it a very suitable model for fundamental studies, and only this type will be discussed further. Table 1 shows the volume, number of cells in the trophectoderm, and total Na, Cl and K in the blastocoele fluid as the rabbit blastocyst develops. All five parameters increase exponentially.

TRANSPORT OF WATER ACROSS THE TROPHECTODERM

Basically, the formation of blastocoele fluid involves the transport of solutes and water across the trophectoderm. Analyses of blastocoele fluid of the rabbit (*Hafez*, 1971) show that the most abundant molecular species is water, and therefore the expansion of the blastocyst is caused primarily by the accumulation of this compound.

In 1970 *Tuft* and *Böving* postulated that water is actively transported across the trophectoderm into the blastocoele. This suggestion has been controversial since active transport of water is known to occur only rarely in nature, such as in a few terrestrial arthropods (*Beament*, 1965). *Borland, Biggers*, and *Lechene* (1976) showed that 6-day-old rabbit blastocysts continued to swell when incubated in media in which the chemical potential of water had been lowered by the addition of sucrose. This result, however, should not be used to support the hypothesis of *Tuft* and *Böving* (1970) that water is actively transported into the blastocoele cavity. Significantly, it was shown that the 6-day-old rabbit blastocyst compensated for the presence of sucrose in the bathing medium by the accumulation of extra NaCl in the blastocoele fluid. For every 2 mM sucrose in the external medium, 1 mM Na and 1 mM Cl accumulated. The stoichiometry of this relation strongly suggests that the transport of NaCl across the trophectoderm into the blastocoele cavity is responsible for the coupled transport of water, and that the active transport of water does not occur.

During the past 15 years, two models have been proposed to explain how water is passively moved across epithelial membranes coupled to active ion transport. These are the double-membrane model and the local osmotic standing-gradient model (see *Diamond*, 1977, *Spring* and *Hope*, 1978 for recent reviews). The two models can be distinguished by examining the osmolality of the fluid transported as a function of the osmolality of the external medium. *Borland, Biggers*, and *Lechene* (1977) aspirated the blastocoele fluid from rabbit blastocysts 6 days post-coitum and allowed them to re-expand over 24 hr in media whose osmolalities ranged from 200–400 mOsmols. At the end of the incubation, samples of the accumulated fluid were obtained by micropuncture and their osmolalities determined with a modified Ramsay-Brown osmometer. The results are shown in Figure 3. There is a clear linear relationship between

Table 1. The Volume, Number of Cells in the Trophectoderm, and Total Na, Cl and K in the Blastocele Fluid at Different Stages of Development of the Rabbit Blastocyst

Age (days)	Vol (μl)[a]	No. Cells in Trophectoderm (in thousands)[a]	Total Na (nmol)[b]	Total Cl (nmol)[b]	Total K (nmol)[b]
4	0.016	1	2	13	0.11
5	0.57	9	76	46	6
6	11.5	80	1540	1277	111
7	66.1	255	?	?	?
8	345	770	?	?	?

[a] From *Daniel* (1964).

[b] Estimated approximately from the volume and concentrations of Na, Cl and K by *Borland, Biggers*, and *Lechene* (1976).

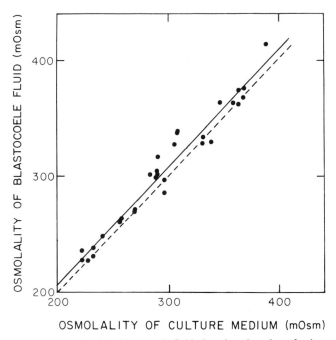

Fig. 3. The osmolality of rabbit blastocoele fluid plotted against that of culture medium. The solid line is the linear regression of the data and has a unit slope. The dashed line represents isosmotic fluid transport. The displacement of the solid line from the dashed line is significant (P = 0.002) and indicates slightly hypertonic fluid transport. From *Borland*, *Biggers*, and *Lechene*, J Reprod Fert 51:131–135, 1977.

the osmolalities of the bathing fluid and the blastocoele fluid that accumulated. Moreover, the fluid which accumulated was slightly hypertonic. This evidence suggests that water is transported across the trophectoderm of the rabbit into the blastocoele cavity according to the local osmotic standing-gradient model.

The development of the local osmotic standing-gradient model was stimulated by attempts to formulate a geometrical basis for the transport of water across epithelial membranes. The essential physiological feature of the local osmotic standing-gradient model is that solutes, e.g., Na^+ and Cl^-, are pumped into a diffusion-restricted compartment such as an intercellular space or the space between microvilli. Recently *Wright*, *Wiedner*, and *Rumrich* (1977), in studies of fluid secretion by the frog choroid plexus, have pointed out that an unstirred layer can also function as a diffusion-restricted compartment. The location of the tight junctions and the presence of lateral intercellular spaces between adjacent cells in the rabbit and mouse trophectoderm provide the necessary anatomical arrangements for the "forward" operation of a standing gradient flow system (*Ducibella et al.*, 1975; *Hastings* and *Enders*, 1975). However, the fact that blastocoele fluid collects in a closed compartment raises the possibility that an unstirred layer may play an important role as well as the intercellular spaces between the trophoblast cells.

ACTIVE NA⁺ TRANSPORT ACROSS THE TROPHECTODERM

The "forward" operation of the local osmotic standing-gradient model requires the presence of active transport systems on the juxtacoelic surface of the trophoblast cells to create the local osmotic gradients in the diffusion-restricted compartments. Evidence already discussed suggests that the Na^+ pump is a likely system. This possibility was suggested by the results of *Smith* (1970), who showed that large concentrations of ouabain in the medium prevent swelling of the rabbit blastocyst and the accumulation of Na^+ and Cl^-.

An important advance was made by *Cross* (1971, 1973), who determined the short-circuit current (I_{sc}) of the trophectoderm of the 6-day-old rabbit blastocyst and the fluxes of Na^+ and Cl^- (Table 2). Since $J_{mb}^{Na^+} > J_{mb}^{Na^+}$ and $J_{mb}^{Cl^-}$, both Na^+ and Cl^- are transported by forces other than those arising from the electrochemical gradient. An estimate of the current due to the transport of Na^+ and Cl^- under short-circuit conditions is:

$$J_{net}^{Cl^-} - J_{net}^{Na^+} = 0.59 - 0.58 = 0.01 \ \mu mol \ cm^{-2} \ h^{-1},$$

which is not significantly different from zero. Thus, the transport of Na^+ and Cl^- may be coupled with only one ion being actively transported. Since the observed I_{sc} was 0.19 $\mu mol \ cm^{-2} \ h^{-1}$, at least one other ionic component is being transported conductively, such as a cation from the blastocoele cavity to the outside, or an anion from the outside into the blastocoele. Replacement of the external medium with HCO_3^--free medium reduced the I_{sc} and this could be reversed by restoring the original medium. Thus, the I_{sc} depends in part on the presence of HCO_3^-.

Table 2.   Unidirectional and Net Na^+ and Cl^- Fluxes ($\mu mol \ cm^{-2} \ hr^{-1}$). Short-circuit Current (I_{sc}) ($\mu mol \ cm^{-2} \ h^{-1}$) and Resistance ($\Omega \ cm^2$) of the 6-day-old Rabbit Blastocyst*

Ion	J_{mb}	J_{bm}	J_{net}	I_{sc}	Resistance
Cl^-	1.73 ± 0.10 (6)	1.14 ± 0.11 (8)	0.59 ± 0.14	0.18 ± 0.01 (14)	2673 ± 164 (14)
Na^+	1.39 ± 0.09 (7)	0.81 ± 0.13 (9)	0.58 ± 0.15	0.20 ± 0.01 (16)	2624 ± 173 (16)

* Results are given as mean ± SEM. Numbers in parentheses represent number of blastocysts observed. From *Cross*, Biol Reprod 8:556–575, 1973.

Table 3.   Components of the Net Ionic Transport and I_{sc} of 6-day-old Rabbit Blastocysts*

Ion	J_{net} (μmol cm^{-2} h^{-1})	Sign of Current
Na$^+$	0.58	−
Cl$^-$	0.59	+
HCO$_3)^-$	0.18	+
Net ionic transport	1.35	—
I_{sc} (μmol cm^{-2} h^{-1})	0.19	—

* Data from *Cross* (1973).

It is instructive to set up a balance sheet by assuming that only Na$^+$, Cl$^-$ and HCO$_3^-$ are the main contributors to the I_{sc} (Table 3). If the blastocyst is 3 mm in diameter, the rate of accumulation of HCO$_3^-$ per blastocyst will be approximately 50 mmol hr^{-1}. This value is identical to the estimate obtained by *Biggers* and *Bellvé* (1974) using totally different assumptions. *Cross* (1974) also measured the rate of accumulation of HCO$_3^-$ by the 6-day-old rabbit blastocyst and found it to be 32 mmol hr^{-1}; this estimate is the same order of magnitude as the estimate obtained by *Biggers* and *Bellvé* (1974), and from the I_{sc}. Thus, the active transport of HCO$_3^-$ into the blastocoele cavity accounts for a significant portion of the I_{sc} of the 6-day-old rabbit blastocyst. Nevertheless, its contribution is only about one-third the contributions of Na$^+$ and Cl$^-$, which are approximately equal but of opposite sign.

The results shown in Table 3 indicate that the net ionic transport of Na$^+$, Cl$^-$ and HCO$_3^-$ is 1.35 μmol cm^{-2} hr^{-1}, while that of Na$^+$ and Cl$^-$ is 1.17 μmol cm^{-2} hr^{-1}. *Borland, Biggers,* and *Lechene* (1977) demonstrated that the 6-day-old rabbit blastocyst accumulates fluid which is 1.03 times isotonic. It can be calculated that in a blastocyst 3 mm in diameter, these net ionic transports could move fluids at the rate of 58.9 and 51.1 μl day^{-1}, respectively. It has been observed that between 6 to 7 days post-coitum, rabbit blastocysts accumulate about 51 μl day^{-1}. This result provides further evidence that the transport of water across the trophectoderm into the blastocoele cavity of the 6-day-old rabbit is determined primarily by the transport of Na$^+$ and Cl$^-$.

The active pump on the juxtacoelic surface of the trophectoderm is probably Na$^+$, K$^+$-ATPase (E.C.3.6.13). Recently *Biggers, Borland,* and *Lechene* (1978) have shown that the microinjection of ouabain into the blastocoele of 6-day-old rabbit blastocysts results in a 13.86 mM rise in K concentration in the blastocoele fluid and concomitant falls in concentrations of 16 mM Na and 10 mM Cl. Exposure of the abcoelic surface of the trophectoderm to ouabain produced no detectable effect.

Also, *Vorbrodt et al.* (1977) were able to demonstrate Na$^+$, K$^+$-ATPase histochemically only in the morula and blastocyst of the mouse in the region of the intercellular spaces between the trophoblast cells.

DEVELOPMENTAL CHANGES IN THE IONIC TRANSPORT SYSTEMS OF THE TROPHECTODERM

Net ionic fluxes also have been estimated from electron probe microanalyses of the elemental composition of the blastocoele fluid and estimates of the rate of fluid transport across the trophectoderm and its surface area. *Borland, Biggers,* and *Lechene* (1976) have used this approach to estimate the net ionic fluxes of Na$^+$, Cl$^-$ and K$^+$ across the trophectoderm of the rabbit at different stages of development (Table 4). The fluxes of Na$^+$ and Cl$^-$ in the 6-day-old rabbit blastocyst obtained by this method, and by radiotracers under short-circuit conditions (Table 3), are of the same order of magnitude. The results in Table 4 show clearly that the rate of transport of all three elements increases markedly from the fourth to sixth days of development.

More recent measurements of the transtrophectoderm potential (ΔV_t) indicate that a more profound developmental change in ion transport occurs in 6- to 7-day-old rabbit blastocysts, shortly before the expected time of implantation (Fig. 4) (*Powers, Borland,* and *Biggers,* 1977). Prior to the sixth day, ΔV_t becomes positive rapidly and attains a mean value of about +21 mV. The potential generated across the epithelium is directly proportional to the resistance of the epithelium and the rate at which ions are moved across. The change in potential which is observed between days 6 and 7 post-coitum may therefore be caused by either an increase in the resistance of the trophectoderm or an increase in the net movement of ions across the barrier.

Figure 5 demonstrates the effect of amiloride on ΔV_t of a 6½- to 7-day-old rabbit blastocyst in a modified F10 medium (*Van Blerkom* and *Manes,* 1974). A concentration of 1 μM caused a slight drop in ΔV_t after

Table 4.   Rate of Transport (μmoles cm^{-2} h^{-1}) of Na, Cl and K in the 4- to 6-day-old Rabbit Blastocyst

	Days post-coitum		
Element	4	5	6
Na	0.098	0.34	0.45
Cl	0.058	0.21	0.36
K	0.005	0.025	0.031

From *Borland, Biggers,* and *Lechene,* Devel Biol 50:201–211, 1976.

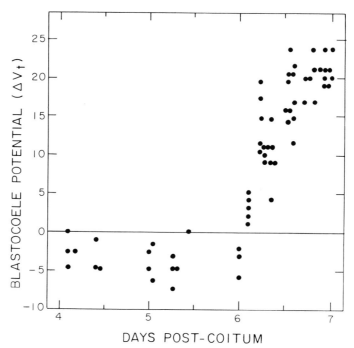

Fig. 4. Developmental changes in the transtrophectodermal potential difference (ΔV_t) measured in freshly collected rabbit blastocysts on days 4,5,6 and 7 post-coitum. From *Powers*, *Borland*, and *Biggers*, Nature 270:603–604, 1977.

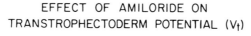

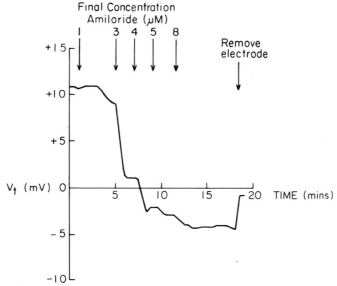

Fig. 5. Effect of different concentrations of amiloride on the transtrophectoderm potential difference (ΔV_t) of the 6½-day-old rabbit blastocyst.

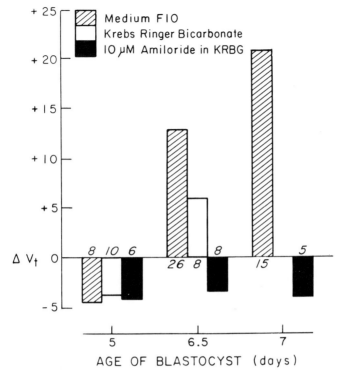

Fig. 6. Mean transtrophectoderm potential (ΔV_t) of 5-, 6.5- and 7-day-old rabbit blastocysts in media with and without 10 μM amiloride. The numbers associated with each block are the number of blastocysts observed. Based on the data of *Powers et al.*, 1977.

a short delay. Raising the concentration to 3 μM caused an immediate rapid reversal of ΔV_t so that it became negative. Other studies showed that a concentration of 10 μM reduced the value of ΔV_t in 6½- to 7-day-old blastocysts to the level characteristic of blastocysts prior to the sixth day of development (Fig. 6). The same concentration of amiloride, however, had no effect on ΔV_t in 5-day-old blastocysts (Fig. 6).

Amiloride has been used extensively to analyze Na transport in several other epithelia and is presumed to act by blocking passive Na entry into epithelial cells (see *Benos* and *Mandel*, 1978 for a review). The effects of amiloride upon the transtrophectodermal potential of the rabbit blastocyst are consistent with the hypothesis that there is an increase in the rate of Na influx across the trophectoderm into the blastocoele.

REFERENCES

Beament, J.W.L. 1965. The active transport of water. Evidence, models and mechanisms. Symp Soc Exp Biol 19:273–298

178   Biggers and Powers

Benos, D.J., and Mandel, L.J. 1978. Irreversible inhibition of sodium entry sites in frog skin by a photosensitive amiloride analog. Science 199:1205–1206

Biggers, J.D. 1972. Mammalian Blastocyst and Amnion Formation. In *The Water Metabolism of the Fetus*, eds. A.C. Barnes and A.E. Leeds, pp. 3–31. Springfield, Ill.: Thomas

Biggers, J.D., and Bellvé, A.R. 1974. Carbon Dioxide in Developmental Processes. In *Carbon Dioxide and Metabolic Regulations*, ed. G. Nahas and K.E. Schaefer, pp. 87–106. New York: Springer Verlag

Biggers, J.D., Borland, R.M., and Lechene, C.P. 1978. Ouabain-sensitive fluid accumulation and ion transport by rabbit blastocysts. J Physiol (Lond) 280:319–330

Borland, R.M., Biggers, J.D., and Lechene, C.P. 1976. Kinetic aspects of rabbit blastocoele fluid accumulation. An application of electron probe microanalysis. Devel Biol 50:201–211

Borland, R.M., Biggers, J.D., and Lechene, C.P. 1977. Fluid transport by rabbit preimplantation blastocysts. J Reprod Fert 51:131–135

Calarco, P.G., and Brown, E.A. 1969. An ultrastructural and cytological study of the preimplantation development in the mouse. J Exp Zool 171:253–284

Cross, M.H. 1971. Rabbit blastocoele perfusion technique. Nature 232:635–637

Cross, M.H. 1973. Active sodium and chloride transport across the rabbit blastocoele wall. Biol Reprod 8:566–575

Cross, M.H. 1974. Rabbit blastocoele bicarbonate accumulation rate. Biol Reprod 11:654–662

Daniel, J.C. 1964. Early growth of the rabbit trophoblast. Amer Nat 98:85–98

Diamond, J.M. 1977. The epithelial junction: Bridge, gate and fence. Physiologist 20:10–18

Ducibella, T., Albertini, D.F., Anderson, E., and Biggers, J.D. 1975. The preimplantation mammalian embryo: Characterization of intercellular junctions and their appearance during development. Devel Biol 45:231–250

Ducibella, T., Ukena, T., Karnovsky, M. and Anderson, E. 1977. Changes in cell surface and cortical cytoplasmic organization during early embryogenesis in the preimplantation mouse embryo. J Cell Biol 74:153–167

Hafez, E.S.E. 1971. Some maternal factors affecting physiochemical properties of blastocysts. In *The Biology of the Blastocyst*, ed. R.J. Blandau, pp. 139–191. University of Chicago Press

Hastings, R.A., and Enders, A.C. 1975. Junctional complexes in the preimplantation rabbit embryo. Anat Rec 181:17–34

Hillman, N., Sherman, M.I., and Graham, C. 1972. The effect of spatial arrangement on cell determination during mouse development. J Embryol Exp Morph 28:262–278

Izquierdo, L., Fernandez, S., and Lopez, T. 1976. Cell membrane and cell junctions in differentiation of preimplanted mouse embryos. Arch Biol Med Exper 10:130–134

Lewis, W.H., and Gregory, P.W. 1929. Cinematography of living developing rabbit eggs. Science 69:226–229

Nilsson, O. 1967. Attachment of rat and mouse blastocysts onto uterine epithelium. Int J Fert 12:5–13

Powers, R.D., Borland, R.M., and Biggers, J.D. 1977. Amiloride-sensitive rheogenic Na^+ transport in rabbit blastocyst. Nature 270:603–604

Schlafke, S., and Enders, A.C.   1967.   Cytological changes during cleavage and blastocyst formation in the rat. J Anat 102:13–32

Smith, M.S.   1970.   Active transport in the rabbit blastocyst. Experientia 26:736–738

Spring, K.R., and Hope, A.   1978.   Size and shape of the lateral intercellular spaces in a living epithelium. Science 200:54–58

Tarkowski, A.K., and Wroblewska, J.   1967.   Development of blastomeres of mouse eggs isolated at the 4- and 8-cell stage. J Embryol Exp Morph 18:155–180

Tuft, P.H., and Böving, B.G.   1970.   The forces involved in water uptake by the rabbit blastocyst. J Exp Zool 174:165–172

Van Blerkom, J., and Manes, C.   1974.   Development of preimplantation rabbit embryos, II. A comparison of qualitative aspects of protein synthesis. Devel Biol 40:40–51

Vorbrodt, A., Konwinski, M., Solter, D., and Koprowski, H.   1977.   Ultrastructural cytochemistry of membrane bound phosphatase in preimplantation mouse embryos. Devel Biol 55:117–134

Wright, E.M., Wiedner, G., and Rumrich, G.   1977.   Fluid secretion by the frog choroid plexus. Exp Eye Res Suppl 25:149–155

Index